LIVING WITH CHRONIC SINUSITIS

LIVING WITH CHRONIC SINUSITIS

The Complete Health Guide to Preventing and Treating Colds, Nasal Allergies, Rhinitis and Sinusitis

DAVID W. KENNEDY, MD, FACS

AND MARILYN OLSEN

healthylivingbooks

New York • London

LIVING WITH CHRONIC SINUSITIS

Healthy Living Books
Hatherleigh Press
5-22 46th Avenue, Suite 200
Long Island City, NY 11101
www.healthylivingbooks.com

DISCLAIMER
This book does not give legal or medical advice.
Always consult your doctor, lawyer, and other professionals.
The names of people who contributed anecdotal material have been changed.

Names of medications are typically followed by TM or ® symbols, but these symbols are not stated in this book.

The ideas and suggestions contained in this book are not intended as a substitute for consulting with a physician. All matters regarding your health require medical supervision.

Library of Congress Cataloging-in-Publication Data

Kennedy, David W., 1948-
  Living with chronic sinusitis / David W. Kennedy.
      p. cm.
  Includes bibliographical references and index.
  ISBN 1-57826-103-1
  1. Sinusitis--Popular works. I. Title.
  RF425.K46 2004
  616.2'12--dc22

                                    2004011233

All Hatherleigh Press titles are available for bulk purchase, special promotions, and premiums. For information about reselling and special purchase opportunities, please call 1-800-528-2550 and ask for the Special Sales Manager.

Cover and interior design by Deborah Miller

10 9 8 7 6 5 4 3 2 1
Printed in Canada

DEDICATION

TO MY PATIENTS: I dedicate this book to you because I have learned so much about this disease as we have managed it together. The practice of medicine is a privilege, and I have learned from your observations, insights, and helpful comments. I am also very grateful for the donations for research within the field that many of you have provided. This research is helping us further our understanding of this common problem.

TO THE HEALTH CARE PROFESSIONALS WHO WORK WITH ME: I dedicate this book to you because, without your dedication and caring, we would not have been able to improve the quality of so many peoples' lives. Christine Reger, CRNP, Kathy Pirolli, RN, Jeanette Gonzales, and my residents and fellows: Thank you.

CONTENTS

INTRODUCTION

S INUSITIS (ALSO CALLED RHINOSINUSITIS) IS NOTHING TO sneeze at. Each year, in the United States alone, more than 37 million sufferers have at least one attack. A much smaller, but still very significant, number of people go on to have chronic and recurrent problems with sinusitis. In this group, sinusitis can become a disorder that seriously affects their overall enjoyment of life and, in some, even their ability to function well on a day-to-day basis.

Most sinus infections result initially from colds. While there's still no cure for colds, there is a lot that can be done to control the symptoms of sinusitis and, through education and medication, also reduce the chances that it will become a chronic and debilitating problem.

That's not to say it's always easy. Inflammation in the sinuses may be brought on by one of the most frequent things we humans do— breathe. Additionally, those who suffer from sinusitis may have no alternative but to be around the things that bother them the most— pollution, pollen, smoke, animal dander, dust, mold, and the many natural and synthetic materials that surround us all every day.

Although sinusitis is common, there is still a lot that we do not know about why it becomes chronic in some people and may develop into an almost disabling disease with a major impact on their quality of life. Fortunately, in the past 20 years we have learned much more about it, what can be done to keep it becoming chronic, and how to treat it when it does not respond to the usual solutions.

Although millions of people suffer from sinusitis, it still remains a very individual problem. Environmental issues that cause irritation are not the same in every person. A person may be born with a predisposition toward sinusitis, whereas another person develops it after an accident or surgery that changes the dynamics of his or her nose.

About 30 years ago, as we began to use small endoscopes to see into the nose and sinuses, and as CT scans became more readily available, we started to see and identify this disease more accurately. I became intrigued with the problem because I knew that many of the treatments that had been used up to that point were not working well. For the first time, we could really study the problem and see why the disease persisted, and also observe why some treatments worked and others did not.

For the past 20 years, I have limited my practice to the medical management and surgery of sinus disease. As a result of what I have learned, I have gained a better understanding of this sometimes difficult problem. In most cases medical management can resolve sinusitis; however, for those cases in which it does not, I introduced a new and less invasive form of surgery into the United States. I termed this technique Functional Endoscopic Sinus Surgery. In situations where medical therapy does not work, this has now become the standard surgical approach worldwide.

I became fascinated with studying the problem of sinusitis in all of its different manifestations and, because sinusitis is so widespread and so little was known about it, I have had the opportunity to teach hundreds of courses to physicians throughout the world, as well as to publish widely in the field. One of the most interesting things that I noted early on was how ubiquitous this disease is. Whether I was getting off an airplane in another city or another country, the physician meeting me would often say, "You have come to the right place, this is the sinus capital of the world!"

Wherever in the world it occurs, one of the most important aspects for living with sinusitis is that those who suffer from it know as much as possible about the disease. Because so many people have problems with sinusitis, there is now a dizzying array of products that claim to offer relief. Before you spend a lot of time and money on any of them, though, you owe it to yourself to discover just what it is that causes you to suffer and which of the many options is actually likely to work for you.

Although sinusitis is initially the result of an infection, the treatments that work best at first—such as antibiotics—don't continue to work in the long run, particularly if the bacteria in your body develop a resistance to them. Sometimes, too, the best solution can be the easiest and even the cheapest, like avoiding smoke or other irritants or using salt water or steam. Additionally, new medications coming into the market offer alternative, but sometimes very expensive, approaches to this problem.

Despite the many committees that I have served on, the hundreds of papers I have written, and the thousands that I have read, there is still an enormous amount that we do not know about this common but sometimes stubborn, and occasionally disabling, disease. Why does it behave so differently in different people? Why do some treatments and drugs work very well for some people, but not well at all for others? Why doesn't surgery—even as sophisticated as it now is—work as well as simple home remedies?

What I do know, however, is that the patients who know the most about their disease, generally have the best chance of finding treatments that work the best for them. That is why I think this book will help you. The information in it is based on the questions most frequently asked by my patients. The suggestions range from the most basic things you can do at home at very little cost or inconvenience to the newest and most scientifically advanced therapies and surgeries now available. Whether you only have a sinus infection once every few years or suffer from its symptoms day in and day out for months at a time, I hope and believe you will find the information that follows useful.

Sinusitis is common, but it needn't be as much of a nuisance as it is for most people. Hopefully, this book will show you how you can prevent and treat both yourself and your family now and in the years to come.

David W. Kennedy, MD
2004

1

WHAT IS SINUSITIS?

An Introduction to Sinusitis, Rhinitis, and Rhinosinusitis

AT SOME TIME OR ANOTHER, ALMOST EVERYONE suffers from a combination of symptoms that include a runny nose, dull headache, and feeling of pressure behind the eyes. For most people, these turn out to be symptoms of the common cold. For others, however, the problem may be—or may soon develop into—a condition known as sinusitis or rhinosinusitis. (The terms are used mostly interchangeably throughout the book.)

Rhinosinusitis is far from rare. If all age groups and different manifestations of the disease are considered, it may be the most common health care complaint in the United States today. It is estimated that more than 37 million Americans suffer from at least one episode of acute rhinosinusitis each year and, as the world becomes increasingly filled with air pollution and other toxins (as with the increasing incidence of asthma), that number is growing. Rhinosinusitis is so widespread it is estimated that, on average, Americans miss four days of work a year due to discomfort produced by the condition. For many people, sinusitis may just be an annoyance but, for others, it can become a chronic problem severely affecting their overall quality of life. However, because the onset of chronic sinusitis is often insidious and slow, the deterioration of the quality of life may not be fully recognized by the patients themselves, let alone by the physicians who treat them. According to the Center for Disease Control's National Center for Health Statistics, 16.3 percent of people older than 18 years of age have rhinosinusitis. Rates appear to be the highest among women and people living in the South. Unlike many of the parts of the body, the sinuses don't fully develop until around age 20 but, nonetheless, sinusitis is a disease that can strike people of any age. Every year, doctor visits for rhinosinusitis total more than 11.7 million; hospital outpatient visits total about 1.2 million. Direct health care costs for rhinosinusitis in the United States have been estimated at six billion dollars annually, and this figure does not include all the time lost from work and decreased work productivity associated with the disorder.

Unfortunately, since people are often unaware that what they have is rhinosinusitis, many spend a good deal of money and time attempting to treat the symptoms with medicines and procedures that not only do not help, but may actually allow their rhinosinusitis to become worse. Unlike a cold, treatment for bacterial rhinosinusitis usually requires attention by a health care provider, and often a prescription antibiotic as well.

For many years, rhinitis and sinusitis were thought to be separate conditions. Rhinitis was considered a disease of the nose, sinusitis a disease of the sinus cavities. However, since the mid-1990s, physicians have come to understand that, since the mucous membranes of the nose and sinuses are continuous and are subject to many of the same problems, the two conditions are typically one and the same. Hence, we have come to believe that the term rhinosinusitis is a more accurate way to describe the condition. In 1996, the American Academy of Otolaryngology–Head, and Neck Surgery established specific criteria for describing the subtypes of the disease, which have now been widely accepted by researchers, physicians, and other health care professionals.

Simply put, rhinosinusitis is an inflammation in the membrane that lines any of the nasal sinuses, the cavities that lie within the cheekbones near the eyes. When the mucous membranes in the nasal cavity become swollen, mucus backs up and bacteria can invade the area. Since air can't enter the sinuses and the mucus is unable to drain from them, bacteria have the perfect environment in which to grow and multiply. In this situation, the mucus becomes pus (a liquid composed of white blood cells, bacteria, and cellular debris) and the inflammation is further worsened.

In acute or short-term rhinosinusitis, obstruction of the sinus and the typical absorption of air may lead to the formation of a vacuum within the sinus, which creates the so-called "sinus headache." When one sinus becomes infected, the infection can easily spread to adjoining sinuses. Thus, nearly half of all people suffering from rhinosinusitis have an inflammation or infection in more than one sinus cavity.

Since open sinuses are required for the sensation of normal nasal breathing, patients with obstructed sinuses often sense that they have an obstruction. Additionally, inflammation within a sinus can cause swelling on the same side of the nose, further adding to the feeling of nasal obstruction.

Bacterial rhinosinusitis is usually preceded by a cold (or viral rhinosinusitis), allergy attack (allergic rhinosinusitis), or irritation caused by pollutants. Fortunately, rhinosinusitis is seldom, if ever, fatal. However, because of the close proximity of the sinuses to the brain and central nervous system and the fact that the sinuses are part of the respiratory system, if left untreated, rhinosinusitis can lead to serious complications. While most people recover from rhinosinusitis with few, if any, lasting effects, rhinosinusitis can be a serious threat to people with asthma, cystic fibrosis, or compromised immune systems, such as people with HIV/AIDS.

Allergic rhinosinusitis may be seasonal; that, is a person may experience it only in the fall or spring in reaction to plants that produce pollen at that time. Other people experience allergic rhinosinusitis all year-round, often due to such irritants as dust, mold, mites, environmental pollutants, chemicals, animal dander, or feathers.

Although rhinosinusitis is characterized by fairly specific symptoms, not everyone experiences it in the same way or for the same duration. Fortunately, what most people get is acute rhinosinusitis, a short-term condition that responds well to medication and/or other treatments. Its symptoms usually last up to three weeks. Others, however, may have recurrent or subacute rhinosinusitis consisting of several acute attacks within a year or so. Still others develop chronic rhinosinusitis. These people may experience symptoms for longer than three weeks—sometimes up to a month or more—or their rhinosinusitis may even last for months at a time, or even years.

People with asthma are particularly prone to chronic rhinosinusitis, and people who are allergic to dust, mold, and pollen may also be affected. Symptoms of chronic rhinosinusitis may be less noticeable than those of acute sinusitis, but may be more serious. Fortunately, damage to the sinuses from an acute sinus infection generally heals with no lasting harm or side effects. However, chronic rhinosinusitis may result in changes within the sinuses or in the regions adjacent to the sinuses, which may require surgery to correct.

What Are the Sinuses?

From a strictly scientific viewpoint, sinuses are any hollow cavities in the body, including the channels for venous blood. In this book, however, we will be focusing on the sinuses that are hollow air spaces located in the head, and which surround the nose, known more specifically as the paranasal sinuses. They include the frontal sinuses over the eyes in the eyebrow area, the maxillary sinuses located inside the cheekbones, the ethmoid sinuses located behind the bridge of the nose between the eyes, and the sphenoid sinuses located behind the ethmoid sinuses in the upper nose area behind the eyes.

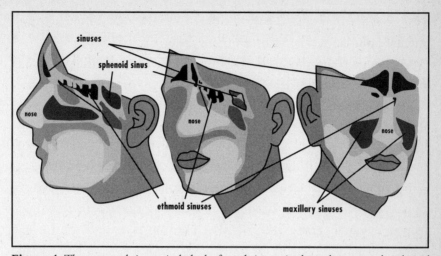

Figure 1. *The paranasal sinuses include the frontal sinuses in the eyebrow area, the ethmoid sinuses between the eyes, the sphenoid sinuses located behind the ethmoid sinuses and behind the eyes, and the maxillary sinuses inside the cheekbones.*

How Do the Sinuses Work?

The sinuses are located within the bones of the face and head. They are lined with four types of ephthelial cells: ciliated columnar epithelial cells, nonciliated columnar cells, basal cells, and goblet cells. The first layer contains somewhere between 50 and 200 cilia (tiny hairs) per cell that beat up to 800 times a minute and move the mucus in the sinuses along. The nonciliated cells contain microvilli (minute structures on the surface of the cell) that increase the surface area of the sinus cavity and help to both increase the humidity of the air in the sinus cavity and warm it. The goblet cells produce glycoproteins, which make the mucus viscous and elastic. It is not yet known what the basal cells do.

Beneath the epithelial layer is a thin membrane where the mucinous glands (that produce mucus) are located. The cilia move this mucus out of the sinus cavities and into the nose. When we breathe, the "mucus blanket" in the nose efficiently traps dirt and other debris.

This mucus, with its entrapped dirt, bacteria, and pollen, is then moved backward by the cilia into the throat. From here it is swallowed, and the acids in the stomach render harmless both the particles and the bacteria on the mucus.

The sinuses are connected to the nose by a continuous layer of mucous membrane. Each sinus opens into the nose and is designed in such a way, that in an ideal situation, air and mucus flow easily between the two. Although we often think of mucus as an unpleasant thing, mucus is very important to our health and well being. Composed of mucins (glycosylated proteins) and inorganic salts suspended in water, mucus coats the cells that line the nose and sinuses and serves the important role of lubricating membranes and protecting them from harmful substances like smoke, dirt, air pollution, and the host of other things we regularly breathe into our noses every day. It also contains substances that are active against both bacteria and viruses (immunoglobulins and defensins). Mucus is also a component of saliva and coats the respiratory, gastrointestinal, and genital tracts.

The sinuses are part of the upper respiratory tract, which also includes the larynx (voice box), pharynx (the part of the throat between the tonsils and the larynx), and connects to the lower respiratory tract (the windpipe or trachea, the bronchial air tubes and the lungs). The sinuses serve several purposes. Since they are filled with air, they make the skull lighter. They also create a "collapse zone" that may help protect the brain in the same way an air bag protects passengers in an automobile. The air-filled sinuses also have a significant effect on the quality of our voices, increasing resonance much like the cavities built into stringed instruments and drums.

However, the major function of the sinuses is to provide the mucus blanket that allows the nose to act as a very effective air conditioner. In addition to providing a sticky surface for the deposition of inhaled particles and bacteria, the mucus secreted by the sinuses provides humidification when dry air is inhaled. No matter how dry the inhaled air, it is almost completely saturated with moisture by the time it reaches the larynx (voice box). Although we are not generally aware of it, when the sinuses are working normally, as much as a quart or more of mucus may be drained through the sinuses each day. Recent studies have shown that the sinuses also produce nitrous oxide, a gas that is toxic to some bacteria, fungi, and viruses.

Ordinarily, the sinuses are sterile, that is, they contain no infections or other microorganisms. Thus, most of the time they remain filled only with air. It is only when either the ostia (the openings into the sinuses)

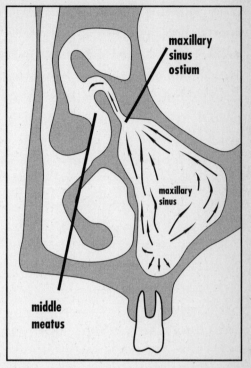

Figure 2. *Tiny hairs called cilia beat up to 800 times a minute to move mucus in the sinuses up along the walls and out through the sinus ostium, clearing the sinuses and nose of dirt, bacteria, pollen, and the many other things we breathe in every day.*

become blocked, or when the lining becomes very swollen from inflammation, irritants, or allergy exposure, that the cilia can no longer work well and rhinosinusitis occurs.

In the following chapters we will discuss what happens when a person develops rhinosinusitis. We'll examine its causes, symptoms, how it is best diagnosed, and what the options are regarding medication, surgery, and lifestyle changes that can help prevent it. We will end this book with a look at some of the latest treatments that may soon be available

Rhinosinusitis is not a new disease. People have been suffering from it for thousands of years. However, it is becoming significantly more common. Fortunately, today, with prompt diagnosis and conscientious attention, it is a disease that is very treatable and, in most cases, causes few side effects and no lasting harm. If left undiagnosed and untreated, however, rhinosinusitis can lead to serious complications. It can also adversely affect a person's ability to enjoy normal day-to-day activities. Hopefully, this book will help you better understand the disease that you share with millions of people worldwide and learn to manage more effectively with fewer symptoms.

2

ABOUT THE SINUSES
Basic Anatomy

OST PEOPLE DEVELOP FOUR PAIRED PARANASAL sinuses. These are: the frontal sinuses, located over the eyes behind the eyebrows; the ethmoid sinuses, located behind the bridge of the nose between the eye sockets; the sphenoid sinuses, located behind the ethmoid sinuses and behind the eyes; and the maxillary sinuses, located inside the cheekbones. We are only born with two pairs, the maxillary and ethmoid sinuses. The others develop as we grow, although none of our sinuses are fully mature until we reach our late teens or early twenties.

The sinuses develop as extensions arising from the nasal cavity, and their size and the extent to which they develop may vary widely from individual to individual. Generally, if a person has a lot of problems with early childhood infections, the sinuses don't develop completely. In fact, by the time they reach adulthood, about 15 percent of people have failed to develop one or more of them. Fortunately, the absence of one or more sinuses doesn't usually cause any measurable problems to the people who don't have them.

As we discussed in Chapter 1, the sinuses perform several important tasks. They produce mucus, increase the humidity and temperature of the air we breathe, filter out toxins and bacteria, lighten the weight of the skull, provide a cushion in our facial bones, and help our voices resonate. In many animals, the sinuses are lined with olfactory cells, allowing them to have a keener sense of smell than humans. Human sinuses, however, are not part of our olfactory system.

Frontal Sinuses

The frontal sinuses are located in the forehead and over the eyes, right behind the eyebrows. Since the frontal bone in the nose is still membranous at birth, the frontal sinus doesn't usually develop into a bony structure until around age two. The frontal sinuses begin to grow at age five and achieve full size by the late teens. When fully developed, these sinuses are usually not the same size; they also vary widely in size from one person to another. One important issue with the frontal sinuses is their proximity to the brain, which sometimes allows an infection in the sinus to spread to the covering of the brain (meningitis) or into the brain itself (brain abscess). The frontal sinuses are connected to the ethmoid sinuses, and mucus produced in the frontal sinuses usually drains through the ethmoid sinuses into the nasal cavity. Inflammation of the frontal sinuses typically produces pain, and sometimes tenderness, over the eyes.

Maxillary Sinuses

The maxillary sinuses are located inside the cheekbones. These two triangular-shaped sinuses are moderately developed at birth and become larger when the milk teeth (deciduous teeth) descend into the mouth. They experience a second increase in size between ages seven to twelve in conjunction with the development of the permanent teeth. Because of their proximity to some of the teeth, infection in the maxillary sinuses may feel like a pain in the cheek or a toothache.

The maxillary sinuses drain through a relatively narrow passage and an ostium (opening) into the nose. In approximately 30 percent of people evaluated for rhinosinusitis, a second opening into the maxillary sinus (accessory ostium) is found. We think that this second opening is a perforation caused by an earlier infection, in much the same way as a middle ear infection may cause a long-term perforation in the eardrum. Fortunately, accessory ostia rarely cause any problems with the functioning of the sinuses.

The infraorbital nerve (which supplies sensation to the cheek) runs along the side of the maxillary sinus and is one reason why an infection in the maxillary sinuses may create pain in the cheek. Interestingly, the opening of the maxillary sinus is not at the floor of the sinus as one might expect, given that its primary function is to drain mucus from the sinus. Instead, the opening or ostium is at the top of the sinus, and the mucus drains upward as a result of the action of the cilia, into narrow channels known as the ostiomeatal complex (OMC). Having the opening at the top of the sinuses clearly illustrates that the drainage of the sinuses is an active process of mucociliary clearance and not the result of gravity. The OMC, the channel into which the frontal and maxillary sinuses drain, lies in close relationship to the ethmoid sinuses and the middle turbinate, a bony projection on the wall of the nose.

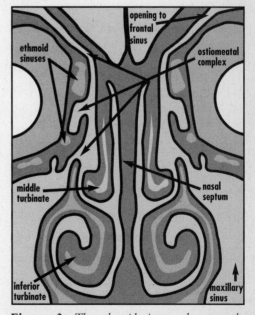

Figure 3. *The ethmoid sinuses closest to the front of the nose and the adjacent nasal structure (the middle turbinate) compose the ostiomeatal complex through which the frontal and maxillary sinuses drain.*

Ethmoid Sinuses

The ethmoid sinuses are located behind the bridge of the nose between the eye sockets. Each ethmoid sinus is composed of from six to twelve small cavities (sometimes up to eighteen) and, like the maxillary sinuses, is fairly well developed at birth. The ethmoid sinuses also continue to grow and reach their adult size around age twelve. The ethmoid sinuses vary considerably in structure. In fact, it is thought that each person's ethmoids may be as distinctive as fingerprints. Ethmoid sinuses have their own ostia that lead into the nasal cavity. The ethmoid sinuses are separated from the orbital cavity that contains the eyes by a very thin bone called the lamina papryacea. Thus, an infection in the ethmoid sinuses may feel like an ache or pressure between the eyes. However, the most common symptoms of ethmoid sinusitis are nasal congestion, nasal discharge, and a feeling of difficulty breathing through the nose. The top of the ethmoid sinuses form the floor of the anterior cranial fossa, the bony structure that separates the sinuses from the frontal lobes of the brain.

The ethmoid sinuses closest to the front of the nose and the adjacent nasal structure (the middle turbinate) make up the OMC. The name—ostiomeatal complex—was given to this area because the frontal and maxillary sinuses drain through it, not through simple openings (ostia) or through straight canals, but via a tortuous course in close relationship to the ethmoid cells themselves. Actually, the maxillary and frontal sinuses drain *between* the ethmoid cells. It is important to understand this relationship because inflammation or infection in the ethmoid sinuses may quickly affect maxillary and frontal sinus drainage.

Sphenoid Sinuses

The sphenoid sinuses are located behind the ethmoid sinuses in the area of the upper nose behind the eyes (just above the nasopharynx). In fact, they lie almost in the center of the head. When fully mature, they are the size of a large grape. The sphenoid sinuses are located adjacent to one another, separated by a thin piece of bone called a septum. Barely visible at birth, they develop from the nasal capsule of the embryonic nose and remain undeveloped until around age three. Like the maxillary sinuses, they begin to grow at age seven and become fully mature in the late teens. Because of the position of the sphenoids, an inflammation in these sinuses cannot only cause pain behind the eyes, but also pain on top or in the back of the head.

The sphenoid sinuses have some important structures close to them. Clearly, they lie close to the brain. The optic nerve (the nerve that carries vision from the eye), the carotid artery (the main blood vessel supplying blood to the brain), and the cavernous sinus (the main vein) run beside the sphenoid sinuses. Hence, an infection in the sphenoid sinuses can sometimes spread to these structures. The nerves that move the eyes (occulomotor nerves) also lie close to these sinuses and occasionally an infection or tumor within the sinus can cause double vision, reduced eye motion or even loss of vision.

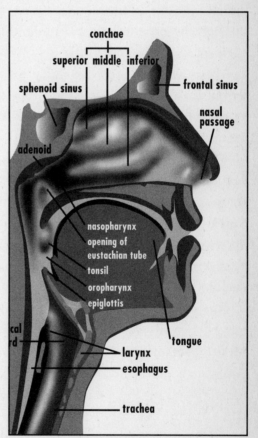

Figure 4. *The sinuses are linked directly to the mouth, nose, and throat by a continuous mucous membrane. Because of this, infections that start in one area, such as in the sinuses, can easily spread to other parts of the upper respiratory system.*

The Nose

Since the sinuses are linked directly to the nose by a continuous mucous membrane, it is also important to understand how the nose is constructed and how what goes on in the nose affects each of the sinuses.

The nose is the uppermost structure in the respiratory system. All air that enters the body does so by way of the nose or mouth. Although it is certainly possible to breathe only through the mouth, from a health standpoint, it is generally best to try to breathe through the nose for reasons we will discuss below. Interestingly, unlike many adults, babies breathe almost exclusively through the nose. In fact if an infant's nose is not open, they will not be able to feed normally.

The nose warms and humidifies the air we breathe and helps filter out bacteria, dirt, pollen, and airborne toxins. It is a very effective air conditioner. And it serves the additional function of being the organ that facilitates the sense of smell.

The tip of the nose is flexible and made of cartilage. The upper portion of the nose, often referred to as the bridge of the nose, is composed of bone. The bottom of the nasal cavity is formed by the hard palate, that is, the portion of the roof of the mouth closest to the front teeth. The nasal cavity ends at the soft palate, which is located at the back of the roof of the mouth where the nose opens into the nasopharynx.

The top of the inside of the nose contains tiny perforations that transmit sensory fibers to the olfactory bulbs located in the brain. Most organic matter releases chemicals, called odorants, by evaporation. (Such inorganic materials as metal or minerals don't release these chemicals and hence have no odor.) The olfactory nerves located in the olfactory bulbs contain receptors (sensory nerve cells) that transmit information about the odors to the brain. The brain then matches this information with what has been stored in the memory, allowing us to distinguish between, for example, the scent of fresh coffee brewing and the scent of a rose. This is a very important function because, in addition to allowing us to recognize pleasurable scents, the brain also can help us identify those that warn us a substance may be harmful (for example, the scent of smoke or leaking gas). Although humans can recognize thousands of separate odors, in comparison to other animals our sense of smell is very weak, causing us to rely to a greater extent on our other senses to identify what is happening around us.

There are a number of reasons why we can lose our sense of smell. However, since it is always necessary for air carrying the odors to reach the olfactory mucosa if a smell is to be perceived, swelling or inflammation of the nasal lining is often one of the causes. About 95 percent of our ability to taste is tied to our ability to smell. So it is little wonder that a stuffy nose affects not only our sense of smell but also our sense of taste.

The nose is divided into two cavities by a piece of cartilage called the nasal septum. The openings of the nose are called the nostrils, or nares, and lead backward into these two cavities. The side wall of the nose, called the lateral nasal wall, is composed of three rounded projections called the superior, middle, and inferior turbinates (also sometimes called conchae). These bony structures, covered with mucous membranes, extend the length of the nasal cavity and act as baffles, directing the passage of air in a winding pattern through the nose rather than in a straight path. The turbinates also increase the surface area of the nose, allowing the air to be warmed further by the blood circulating through the walls of the nose before the air is taken into the lungs. When blood enters the walls of the nose, it also narrows the passageway and gives the turbinates more time to warm the air. When the turbinates detect cold air, they swell and also produce more mucus, which is why our noses run more on cold days.

The space between each turbinate is called a meatus. The sinuses drain mainly into the space between the middle meatus and the side wall of the nose.

The inferior turbinate, the largest of the turbinates, is parallel to the bottom of the nose, and receives the tears that are drained into it

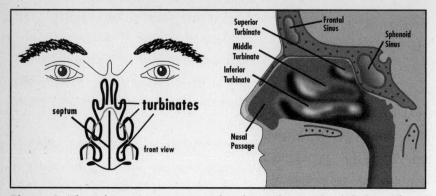

Figure 5. *The turbinates are structures within the nasal cavity that help humidify and filter air as it passes through the nose. The turbinates are also known as concha.*

by the nasolacrimal duct located just below the eyebrow (we will learn more about the structure of the eye later in this chapter). That is why when we cry, we also get a runny nose.

The middle turbinate is located above the inferior turbinate. The ethmoid and maxillary sinuses open into the middle meatus. The frontal sinus also drains into the middle meatus through a funnel-shaped opening called the infundibulum.

The superior turbinate (the smallest turbinate) is located above the middle turbinate. The ethmoid sinuses drain into the superior meatus. Between the superior turbinate, the septum, and the sphenoid sinus, is the sphenoethmoid recess. This is where the sphenoid sinuses drain.

The turbinates also help to control the air flow through the nose. Generally, people breathe primarily through one side of the nose while the other side of the nose "rests." This cycling of which side we breathe through at any moment in time is controlled by the turbinates that alternately swell and decongest on one side and then on the other. This "nasal cycle" typically changes every two to six hours but can also be influenced by other factors. If you lie on one side, it is normal for the nose to become congested on the side you are lying on. There is also some evidence that the nasal cycle can be influenced by mental activity. The turbinates can also swell due to other factors such as menstrual cycle, pregnancy, and allergies. When this happens, mucus can collect in the nose and may create an environment in which bacteria can cause an infection.

As you may remember from Chapter 1, the sinuses all secrete mucus, which is moved by the cilia (a process called mucociliary clearance) into the nose. Although we sometimes refer to this process as sinus drainage, that term is misleading, since the mucus does not simply drain by gravity like water running out of a sink, but is instead moved by the cilia into the nose.

The actual amount of mucus produced in the sinuses and the nose may vary both in quantity and consistency. Generally, mucus is clear and watery but, if the air drawn into the nose is very dry or infection is present, the mucus may become thick and sticky or yellow or green in color. When mucus changes consistency or becomes irritating to the throat, it is called "postnasal drip."

The mucus produced in the nose and sinuses has only two places to go. It must either be expelled out through the nose, or drain to the back of the nose into the nasopharynx. Most of the mucus that reaches the back of the nose is swallowed and moves through the esophagus to the stomach. In the stomach, stomach acid, essentially hydrochloric acid, kills the bacteria that have been collected in the mucus.

The back of the nose is called the nasopharynx. The nasopharynx is connected to the ear by the Eustachian tube. Usually, the Eustachian tube keeps the pressure between the ear and the nose equal but, if the nasopharynx becomes inflamed because of an infection that may have spread from the sinuses or the nose, it may feel like the ears are clogged.

The Ears

The ears can be thought of as sinuses containing air, which have become modified for hearing. In addition to enabling us to hear, of course, our ears also help us maintain our balance.

The ears are divided into three sections: the outer, middle, and inner ear.

The outer ear, the skin-covered cartilage connected to the side of the head, is called the pinna. Although the shape of the pinna is very individual, varying considerably from person to person, the function of the pinna is the same in all people—to collect sound and direct it into the outer ear canal to the eardrum.

The eardrum, also known as the tympanic membrane, is a thin layer of skin that vibrates like a drum when sound reaches it.

The middle ear is composed of three small bones, whose common names correspond to their shape. They are the hammer, anvil, and stirrup. The hammer (the malleus) passes the vibrations from the eardrum to the anvil. The anvil (the incus) passes these vibrations from the hammer to the stirrup. The stirrup (the stapes), which is the smallest bone in the human body, passes the vibrations on to the cochlea, a marvelously engineered organ that amplifies the sound presented to the inner ear.

The cochlea is a spiral-shaped fluid-filled pouch lined with cilia (tiny hairs like those found in the walls of the nose and sinuses). These

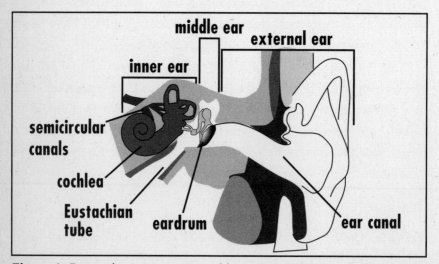

Figure 6. *Because the sinuses are connected by mucous membranes to the ears, untreated sinus infections can spread there, resulting in conditions such as otitis media. An ear infection that causes pain, loss of equilibrium, and sometimes hearing loss, otitis media is more frequently found in children than adults.*

cilia respond to the vibrations received from the middle ear by creating a nerve impulse. This nerve impulse is transmitted to the nerves that carry messages to the brain.

The Eustachian tube connects the middle ear to the back of the nose, somewhat akin to the way the sinuses are connected to the nose. The function of this tube is to equalize pressure between the middle ear and the air pressure outside the body and it opens when someone yawns or chews. When a person rides in an airplane or climbs a mountain, the ears often "pop." This is a sensation created by the body's attempt to balance pressure.

The Eyes

The eyes are amazingly complex structures composed of a network of nerves, blood vessels, fluids, and receptors of various kinds. The parts of the eye that can be seen consist of the iris, pupil, and sclera. The iris is the pigmented portion of the eyeball, that is, it contains the melanin that gives eyes their color. The pupil, in the center of the iris, allows light rays to reach the lens. The lens, composed of proteins and water, focuses the light by muscles that stretch and relax to let more or less light into the eye. The sclera is the "white" of the eye. The purpose of the sclera is to help hold the pupil and lens in place. The clear portion of the sclera is called the cornea. It extends out and over the iris and lens and protects them from dirt, dust, injury, and other irritants.

Behind the visible portions of the eye is the vitreous humor. This is a clear jellylike substance that allows the eye to maintain its shape. At the back of the eye are the retina and macula.

When we look at something, light rays reflect from the object onto the cornea. The cornea focuses the light rays through the lens and vitreous humor onto the retina. The macula works with the retina to focus images in fine detail. As in a camera, the image at this point is upside down. The retina converts the image into electrical impulses that are transmitted through the optic nerve into the brain

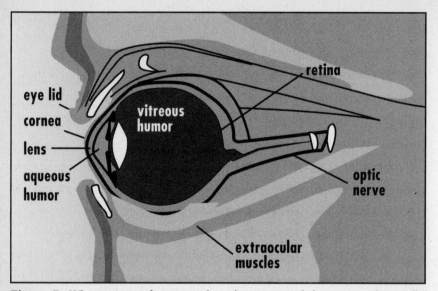

Figure 7. *When a sinus infection spreads to the area around the eye, a condition called orbital cellulitis results. More frequently encountered in children and adolescents than in adults, this disease involves swelling of the eyelids and possibly impaired vision.*

that then analyzes the image and turns it right side up so we can perceive it as it exists in nature.

In addition to receiving and interpreting visual images, the eye also produces tears, whose purpose is to coat the outer surface of the eye, keep it moist, and trap any airborne dust, dirt, or pollutants and keep them from damaging the delicate eye tissues. Tears are composed of oil, water, and mucus and, like nasal secretions, contain chemicals that have antibacterial properties. Every time we blink, the eyelids spread newly formed tears across the surface of the eye and remove old tears. These old tears are pushed into the tiny drains at the corners of the eyelids called puncta, which drain the tears into the upper and lower canaliculus. From there, the tears empty into the lacrimal sac, then into the nasolacrimal duct, and finally into the nose. As we discussed earlier in the chapter, this is why our nose runs when we cry. Additionally, since the lacrimal ducts pass in close proximity to the sinuses, swelling and blockage of the tear duct, with resultant watering of the eye, can sometimes occur as a result of sinus inflammation or, less commonly, sinus tumors.

The Mouth

The mouth serves two major life-sustaining functions. It is the beginning of both the respiratory and digestive systems. Through it, we can take in both air and the nutrients our body needs to function. The mouth also allows us to alter the sounds produced by the vocal cords by changing the shape of the lips and tongue.

The mouth consists of the teeth, the gums, and the tongue.

The teeth are designed to allow us to break pieces of food into portions small enough to swallow without choking. Animals, including humans, have different shapes of teeth depending on the type of food they normally eat. Carnivores (meat eaters) usually have sharper, more pointed teeth in the front of the mouth for tearing flesh. Animals that eat mostly plants have wider, more blunt teeth for grinding up vegetable matter. Humans, being omnivores, that is, animals that eat a variety of foods, have both kinds of teeth.

The tongue is a large and powerful muscle whose main purpose is to move food around in the mouth as the teeth grind the food up, saliva moistens it, and the enzymes in the saliva begin to digest the food prior to sending it into the esophagus. The surface of the tongue is covered with papillae, fine hairs that allow us to "feel" the textures of things in the mouth. Taste buds, located around the tongue allow us to distinguish between flavors that are sweet, salty, sour, or bitter. In addition to allowing us to enjoy the taste of good foods, the taste buds warn us if we are about to swallow something that is rotten or spoiled.

The mouth also produces saliva, which is a liquid composed of water, electrolytes, mucus, and enzymes. Humans have three pairs of salivary glands. The partoid glands produce a watery substance. The submaxillary glands produce mucus, and the sublingal glands secrete saliva that is predominantly mucus. When food enters the mouth, the autonomic nervous system senses the character of the food and produces the appropriate type and amount of saliva.

Saliva performs several functions. It lubricates and binds the food into a ball, called a bolus, that can pass easily through the esophagus. It moistens dry food so we can taste it. Saliva also cleans the mouth by washing away food, bacteria, and other substances so that the breath remains relatively odorless and bacteria don't build up and cause an infection. In addition, the enzymes in saliva start the digestive process and neutralize the acidity in foods. Finally, the saliva cools or heats the food or liquids so that they do not harm the delicate tissues of the esophagus.

The epiglottis is the flap of cartilage located behind the tongue and in front of the opening to the larynx (voice box). Though small, the epiglottis plays a very important role because the respiratory and digestive tracts cross each other in the portion of the throat called the oropharynx. As we swallow, the epiglottis folds back and covers the entrance to the larynx, directing the food into the esophagus and away from the trachea (windpipe). Similarly, the epiglottis relaxes after we swallow, to allow air into the windpipe. The uvula, the fleshy muscle that hangs down from the upper palate, flips up to close off the nasal passages when we swallow. It is very important that excess air not get into the digestive tract or that food not get into the respiratory tract. Excess air in the digestive tract can result in nausea, heartburn, and vomiting. Food that has been aspirated (breathed) into the lungs can cause infections or even death.

The Throat

The upper part of the throat, also known as the pharynx, is the portion of the respiratory system that extends from the back of the nose and mouth to the trachea. Whether we breathe air in through the mouth or the nose, the air will end up in the nasopharynx (the place where the nose and mouth connect) and go from there into the pharynx.

The larynx is located at the top of the trachea. In the larynx, stretched flaps of tissue, called the vocal cords, vibrate and produce sounds.

The throat also contains two structures that can affect and be affected by the sinuses. These are the adenoids and tonsils. The adenoids lie within the nasopharynx about an inch above the uvula. Generally, the adenoids shrink as a child grows. However, sometimes the adenoids remain large and can cause nasal blockage.

The tonsils are clumps of tissue located on either side of the throat next to the soft palate. If you open your mouth very wide you can see the tonsils, but not the adenoids.

Both the tonsils and adenoids are made of lymphoid tissue. Lymphoid tissue is primarily designed to produce antibodies to help fight infections. The adenoids and tonsils are thought to be of importance mainly to infants because they usually shrink or disappear as we mature. Even if they don't shrink, they generally remain harmless. But if the adenoids remain overly large or tend to get infected, they may need to be surgically removed. In addition, tonsils may need to be removed if they become infected constantly. In the past, adenoids and tonsils were removed more often than they are today because now such infections can be treated with antibiotics and generally do not pose as serious a threat as they once did.

3

SYMPTOMS OF SINUSITIS AND RHINITIS
Recognizing Warning Signs

BECAUSE THE SINUSES ARE A PART OF THE respiratory system, it is not surprising that the symptoms of sinusitis are similar to the symptoms of other respiratory diseases. However, even though many of the symptoms may be the same, treatment for various respiratory diseases may be quite different. Therefore, if you experience any of the symptoms listed below, particularly if they are especially unpleasant or persistent for a length of time, it is very important that you see your doctor to find out specifically what the cause of your symptoms may be.

Asthma

Asthma, or reactive airway disease, is a disease of the respiratory system characterized by intermittent airway constriction, causing the sufferer to gasp and wheeze while attempting to breathe. It can occur in children and adults and, if not properly treated, can be dangerous—particularly in children. The incidence of asthma is known to be linked to several other diseases such as environmental allergies, sinusitis, and aspirin allergy, as well as gastroesophageal reflux disease (GERD). In someone who is susceptible, asthma may occur following a cold or flu. If you have asthma or symptoms suggesting asthma, consult your doctor to find out if your asthma symptoms are related to sinusitis.

Cough

A cough may be a symptom of many diseases including sinusitis, a cold, influenza, or GERD (gastroesophageal reflux disease). A persistent cough can also be a manifestation of mild asthma (cough variant asthma) or occasionally can be precipitated by a certain class of medicines used to treat high blood pressure (ACE, or angiotensin-converting enzyme inhibitors). In children, coughing at night is a common symptom of chronic rhinosinusitis. In adults, a persistent cough may also be a symptom of something much more serious such as tuberculosis, Barrett's esophagus (a precancerous condition), or cancer of the throat or lungs. Many smokers or people exposed to airborne toxins may also experience coughing. If a cough persists for more than two weeks, you should see a doctor to determine the exact cause.

Earaches

Earaches can occur in people of all ages, although they are most frequent in young children. In fact, it is estimated that almost all children have at least one ear infection before they reach age seven or eight. These ear infections are usually a condition called otitis media, an infection in the inner ear. Because of the connection between the ears and the sinuses, in both children and adults it may be difficult to know where the infection began. As with sinusitis, otitis media may be acute or chronic and is typically associated with Eustachian tube obstruction. Babies or young children with an earache may exhibit symptoms such as being abnormally fussy, running a fever, pulling on their ears, or placing their hands over their ears.

If the infection is in both ears, they may also experience a temporary loss of hearing. It is important to see a doctor if a child seems to have an earache, because if the infection is not treated, the eardrum may become scarred, and permanent hearing loss and resultant impairment of speech can result. Typically, these infections follow a viral upper respiratory tract infection such as a cold, but the cause of these symptoms could also be sinusitis.

Adults also experience earaches, which may be symptoms of an infection in the ear or in the sinuses. In adults and older children, the symptoms may indicate otitis media (an infection of the inner ear) or otitis externa, an infection in the external ear canal, sometimes called "swimmer's ear."

An extreme earache during air travel, particularly when the air pressure changes rapidly as the plane is taking off or landing, may also be a symptom of a sinus infection or chronic sinusitis. Certainly, it is unwise to fly if you have a cold. Although it happens rarely, Eustachian tube problems can also result in permanent hearing loss if the pressure cannot be equalized as the plane descends.

Fever

When an infection develops, your body has several defenses against it. One is your immune system. Another is to raise the body temperature to a level that will kill the bacteria or viruses that are invading it. Most people maintain a normal body temperature between 97.5 and 101 degrees Fahrenheit. A fever of 102 to 103 degrees may occur with cold or flu symptoms and not necessarily indicate something more serious. However, a fever in an adult above 103 degrees Fahrenheit is generally a symptom that a more severe infection is present. If the fever is combined with pain in the face and/or nasal congestion, the fever may be a symptom of sinusitis.

Headache

Similarly, headaches may be a symptom of several different conditions or diseases ranging from benign to very serious. By far, the most common causes of headache are stress and variations of migraine. However, a headache may also occur with an acute sinusitis. Headache at any time of the day can be a symptom of sinusitis, although it is most often a symptom of sinusitis if it occurs early in the morning.

Itchy and Watery Eyes

Because the tear ducts drain into the sinuses, if an infection is present in the sinuses, it may affect the tissues around the eyes, as well. Although itchy eyes are most often symptoms of seasonal allergies, it is possible that itching may indicate an infection in the sinuses. Persistent watery eyes can be the result of sinusitis or, occasionally, a sinus tumor because the tear duct is positioned close to the sinuses and can be affected by sinus inflammation.

Loss of Smell

As discussed in Chapter 2, tiny perforations inside the nose transmit odorants (chemicals released by organic matter) to the olfactory bulbs in the brain. If the nose or the ethmoid sinuses are congested, these odorants cannot penetrate the congestion. Thus, you have an infection in your sinuses, you may temporarily lose your sense of smell. It is very rare for such a sensory loss to be permanent. However, occasionally it is possible for a viral infection to permanently damage the olfactory nerve. Decreased sense of smell is a common and important symptom of chronic rhinosinusitis. It occurs because of the swelling in the nose, and it usually improves as this is treated. However, prolonged chronic inflammation in the nose can also permanently affect the olfactory system, which may not recover even when the sinusitis is treated.

Nasal Congestion

A lot of air and mucus pass through the sinuses on a daily basis, and this free passage of air is important to your health and sense of well being. When air cannot pass freely, usually you are experiencing nasal congestion, which can be caused by viral infections, allergies, pollutants, septal deviations, or a tumor in the nose. It is also a common symptom of inflamed sinuses.

The sinuses are designed to be filled only with air most of the time and to be open to the nose. If the sinuses become swollen or clogged with mucus due to an infection, the nose feels congested. Chronic sinusitis also has a direct effect on the ability to breathe through the nose because it causes the turbinates in the nose to swell. Turbinate swelling and prolonged nasal congestion are among the more common symptoms of chronic sinusitis.

Nasal Obstruction

Nasal congestion and nasal obstruction are closely related symptoms and, thus, can be difficult to clearly differentiate from each other. Nasal obstruction may be caused by one of several things: a congenital abnormality in the various structures within the nose or sinuses; a misalignment of one of the structures of the nose caused by an injury or, occasionally (particularly when only on one side), a tumor or foreign matter in the nose. However, as mentioned before, nasal obstruction is also a common symptom of sinusitis and the resultant swelling in the nose.

Pain

Pain in various portions of the face or in the teeth can be a symptom of sinusitis. However, severe pain is much more common in acute than chronic sinusitis. When a sinus infection is present, your sinuses may also feel tender to the touch. If the ethmoid sinuses are inflamed, you may experience tenderness and pain along the sides of the nose. A maxillary sinusitis can cause tenderness in the upper teeth. If the frontal sinuses are infected, the forehead may feel tender to the touch or to a gentle tapping with your finger. If the sphenoid sinuses are infected, you may experience pain in the ears, neck, or at the top of the head.

In chronic sinusitis the pain is more typically a dull ache or feeling of pressure, frequently between the eyes, and is usually associated with other symptoms of chronic sinusitis such as discolored discharge and nasal congestion. Although acute sinusitis may cause pain in the forehead, or across the eyebrows and the bridge of the nose (typically described as a "sinus headache"), such headaches are experienced less frequently in chronic sinusitis. Unless they are associated with other sinusitis symptoms, they are more likely to be due to stress, depression or variations of migraine. If you experience severe pain in one of the sinus areas when flying in an airplane (particularly when the aircraft is taking off or descending to land), this can be an important symptom of both chronic or acute sinusitis.

Postnasal Discharge

As we discussed in earlier chapters, the nose and sinuses produce a liter or more of mucus every day, and it has only two places to go—out the nose or down the throat. When the mucus is thin and watery, it drains easily—so easily, in fact, that we barely notice it, even though it is draining continuously. If the mucus becomes infected and the consistency changes, it may be more difficult to swallow and may irritate the lining of the throat and esophagus. This irritation may be a symptom of sinusitis. Postnasal discharge may also be significantly more noticeable in someone with asthmatic tendencies.

Sore Throat

As mentioned above, when the mucus produced by the body becomes infected, it may irritate the lining of the throat. Recurrent sore throats can be a symptom of allergies, chronic sinusitis, or chronic inflammation of the tonsils or adenoids.

Swallowing Problems

Many factors may contribute to difficulty in swallowing (dysphagia), and some of them are very serious, indeed. Difficulty in swallowing, for example, may be a symptom of an enlarged thyroid gland, a neurological problem, or Barrett's esophagus, a precancerous condition caused by acid reflux. Difficulty in swallowing is almost always a symptom that something is wrong with your throat. If you have this symptom, you should see your doctor.

Hoarseness

A hoarse voice is most commonly caused by inflammation of the vocal cords (laryngitis). This condition is usually viral and goes away spontaneously. When hoarseness is prolonged, it can be caused by voice abuse (shouting, singing, and prolonged talking), nodules developing on the vocal cords, or to a variety of other causes such as GERD and allergies. It can also be a symptom of a more severe problem such as a tumor on the vocal cords or in the thyroid gland. Sometimes, hoarseness can result from chronic sinusitis and its associated postnasal drip, resulting in some vocal cord swelling or inflammation. The possibility of chronic sinusitis should, therefore, also be considered when hoarseness is a recurrent symptom. Whatever the cause, hoarseness lasting more than a few weeks should always be evaluated by an otolaryngologist (ear, nose, and throat doctor).

Swelling of the Eyelids

Swelling in the eyelids may be a symptom of sinusitis because the ethmoid sinuses are near the tear ducts in the corner of the eyes, and when these sinuses become inflamed, the eyelids and tissues around the eyes can become swollen or discolored (sometimes called "allergic shiners").

Swollen Lymph Nodes

As we will discuss in Chapter 7, sinusitis may be caused by one of three types of infections: bacterial, viral, or fungal. To combat these invaders, your body contains a sophisticated immune system which operates independently of the system that circulates your blood. This circulates lymph, a transparent fluid that contains the white cells that attack bacteria, viruses, fungi, or any foreign microbes that get into the body. These white cells attempt to destroy the germ before it can multiply and cause a disease. Lymph nodes are located in the groin, neck, underarms, abdomen and, of particular importance for sinusitis sufferers, in the tonsils and adenoids. Lymph tissue is also found in bone marrow (where blood cells are produced), the appendix, the lining of the small intestine, and the spleen. When an infection is present in the body and a battle between the invaders and the lymphocytes is occurring, the lymph nodes often swell and become hard to the touch. If you feel a swollen lymph node, particularly in your neck, it can be a symptom of an infection in your sinuses, or can also reflect other inflammation in the same area. When lymph nodes remain swollen, and particularly if they slowly enlarge, it could be a symptom of cancer or a tumor, and it may be necessary to perform a biopsy.

Tenderness to the Touch

As we discussed earlier in this chapter, although both mucus and air are constantly circulating through the sinuses, most of the time there is only air in the sinuses. If the mucus becomes infected, however, it becomes much thicker in consistency than normal and may not be able to circulate out of the sinus, down the throat to the stomach, or out the nose.

When this occurs, the sinuses become full of mucus and pressure is created. Because some of the sinuses are located near the surface of the face and all are located adjacent to other facial structures, often this pressure can cause pain that can be easily felt if you press your cheeks or jaws.

Tiredness

When your body is experiencing an infection of any kind, you will feel fatigued; this is certainly true of chronic sinusitis. Chronic sinusitis can also affect your sleep, so that you may feel tired during the day. Frequently, chronic sinusitis may be associated with some long-term fatigue although, typically, tiredness is not one of the most marked symptoms.

Toothache

What feels like a toothache, particularly an ache in the upper molar teeth at the back of the mouth may be a symptom of sinusitis. The reason for this is that the maxillary sinuses are located in the bones of the cheeks and when these sinuses are infected, they may exert pressure on the nerves of the teeth.

4

WHEN SHOULD YOU
SEE A DOCTOR?

*When Over-the-Counter
Treatments Don't Work*

ECAUSE SINUSITIS IS SUCH A COMMON
problem and because so many over the counter medications are now available, many people treat their symptoms
without consulting a doctor. Self-diagnosis and treatment
may be appropriate if symptoms are mild and disappear within a few
days. If, however, symptoms are severe or if they persist for more than
just a few days, it is advisable to see a doctor.

As we discussed in the previous chapter, some symptoms are
indicative of more than one illness. A headache, for example, may be
symptomatic of many things, including diseases of the eye or ear,
allergy, pressure on the brain, meningitis and, less commonly, sinusitis.
Because these diseases have different causes, it is important that you
find out what the source of your symptoms may be, so that they can
be treated appropriately. Inappropriate treatment may not only be
expensive and useless in bringing relief to your symptoms but in

some cases, it may actually make your symptoms worse. If you have an infection, for example, and it is not treated appropriately, it may spread to other parts of your body.

What Kind of Doctor Should You See?

Because sinusitis is such a common illness, your family physician has probably seen many patients who have had it. In most cases, your doctor will be able to either recommend nonprescription medications or prescribe a medication such as an antibiotic for you.

If, however, you do not respond to the recommendations made by your family doctor, you may need to see a specialist, probably an otolaryngologist, a doctor who specializes in treating diseases of the head and neck. Otolaryngologists are also sometimes referred to as ENT physicians, that is, physicians who specialize in diseases of the ear, nose, and throat. Otolaryngology is the oldest medical specialty in the United States. All otolaryngologists are trained in the medical and surgical management of diseases and disorders of the sinuses, larynx, mouth, throat, neck and face.

Otolaryngologists complete undergraduate college, four years of medical school, and at least five years of training in their specialty. They must also pass the American Board of Otolaryngology examination in order to be recognized as a specialist in this field. In addition, some otolaryngologists complete one- or two-year fellowships in a subspecialty, which include pediatric otolaryngology (a practice limited to the care of children); otology/neurotology (diseases of the ears and problems with balance and tinnitis or ringing in the ears); allergies; facial plastic and reconstructive surgery; diseases of the head and neck; laryngology (the throat); and rhinology (the nose and sinuses). However, since infections in any part of the head and neck may spread to other areas, otolaryngologists are trained to explore all possibilities before making a specific diagnosis. In this book, we will mention these other specialties briefly, but will be concerned primarily with rhinology.

Why Should I See an Otolaryngologist?

Often, the diagnosis of acute sinusitis is a fairly straightforward one. One of the symptoms described in the previous chapter, pain in the face, for example, may lead the doctor to suspect that you have a bacterial infection in one or more of your sinuses. Your doctor might prescribe an antibiotic and in a few days, the pain and infection are gone.

In other cases, particularly in chronic sinusitis, the diagnosis may not be so simple. The common symptoms of nasal congestion, nasal obstruction, and postnasal discharge may develop gradually over time and be associated with a feeling of pressure, generalized fatigue, poor sleeping, and cough. In this case, the diagnosis may be more difficult, particularly if taking an antibiotic doesn't relieve the symptoms. An otolaryngologist may be helpful in this case because he or she can perform a more detailed examination, including endoscopic examination of the nose, if necessary, and ensure that the most appropriate diagnostic tests are performed. Otolaryngologists can then provide appropriate medical therapy and monitor its efficacy based upon careful examination rather than just symptom improvement. This is an important concept because the two do not necessarily correlate in chronic sinusitis. That is, even though the symptoms may have lessened in severity, the underlying causes of sinusitis may still be present, indicating that the medication or therapy being used might not be working and another medication or therapy may be indicated. Usually, your doctor will ask you questions relating to past illnesses and your current lifestyle, including diet, exercise, medications you take, tobacco and alcohol use, your family, and your job. You should never be embarrassed about what is revealed in these discussions. Whatever you discuss with your doctor remains confidential. Your doctor is not there to make any kind of value judgment about you, only to help you treat your disease. In order to do that effectively, the doctor must understand all the factors that might be contributing to it.

Do I Need to See a Subspecialist in Rhinology?

General otolaryngologists are trained to treat and, when necessary, to perform surgery on sinusitis that does not respond to medical therapy. However, if you have had previous surgery and are still having problems, or if you have an unusual problem (such as a tumor), you may wish to consider being seen by subspecialist in rhinology. A number of the larger cities and major university medical centers in the United States now have fellowship-trained rhinologists. However, the vast majority of sinus disease is still successfully managed by general otolaryngologists.

When Should You Arrive at the Doctor's Office?

You should plan to arrive at the doctor's office at least a half hour earlier than their initial scheduled appointment, since you will need time to fill out your medical history forms. This is a very important process because it will allow the doctor to review pertinent issues about your medical history in an organized manner. You should fill these forms out carefully and accurately as they will likely direct the conversation you will have with the doctor.

What Should You Bring to the Doctor's Office?

Whether you are visiting a family doctor or a specialist, such as an otolaryngologist, it is very helpful to bring along the following:

LIST OF ALL OF YOUR SYMPTOMS
Sometimes what seems like the most insignificant detail is actually the information the doctor needs to make an accurate diagnosis. It is important that the patient remember to tell the doctor not just the primary symptoms, but all symptoms he or she may be experiencing. It is also important to tell the doctor what time of day these symptoms

occur. If possible, you should write all of this information down so that you will not forget any of it during the examination. Below is an example of such a list:

SYMPTOMS:

Nasal congestion: Seems to be worse in the morning, right after I get up. Gets better during the day, but always comes back the next morning.

Cough: Seems to get worse as the day goes on and is the worst at night. Sometimes I wake up during the night coughing.

Pain in my jaw: I have what feels like a toothache in my jaw. I experience the most pain when I am chewing food or gum.

Earache: It also feels like there is pressure in my ears, causing them to "pop" several times during the day.

A concise but complete list like the one above is very important in helping your doctor consider all of your symptoms before making a diagnosis.

LIST OF ALL MEDICATIONS YOU TAKE

As with your list of symptoms, this list needs to be very complete. Many people forget what medicines they are taking or don't think that things like vitamins and herbal supplements are medications. Because a patient has only a limited time with a doctor, it's important that the patient relates to the doctor all his or her medications and supplements, either brings the list or the medications themselves. The list should include:

1. All prescription medications you take.
2. All nonprescription medications you take.
3. All vitamin supplements you take.
4. All herbal medications you take.
5. All food supplements you take.

It is also important that you list the exact quantity you take, when you take it, where you take it, and any activities that you do after you take it. Below is a sample medication list:

Medication	Quantity	Time	Place	What you do next
Aspirin	1 tablet	6 A.M.	Home	eat breakfast
Vioxx	20 MG	6 A.M.	Home	eat breakfast
Forsythia Suspensa	2 capsules	6 A.M.	Home	eat breakfast
Claritin	10 MG	6 A.M.	Home	eat breakfast
Robitussin	1 capful	2 times a day	at work	
Vicks Nasal Spray	1 spray	2 to 3 times a day	at work	
Lipitor	20 MG	10 P.M.	Home	go to bed

As you can see by this sample list, this fictitious patient is taking an aspirin that may have been prescribed as a preventative for cardiac problems, but which could be a factor in sinusitis. The patient is also taking an anti-inflammatory, used primarily in the treatment of arthritis, an herbal medication that is supposed to improve the immune system, an allergy medication, a cough medicine, a nasal spray, and a drug that is used to lower cholesterol. It is very important for a doctor to know that a patient like this is taking all these medications because some of them may actually be aggravating the patient's sinusitis or may be interacting with one another to cause other problems. Additionally, if a surgical procedure is subsequently considered, it is very important for the physician to know if you are taking any herbal supplements or medications that might increase bleeding (such as aspirin, ibuprofen, vitamin E, ginko biloba, and some other herbal medications).

List of All Previous Experience Sinusitis, Sinusitis Medications, or Surgery

In addition to the list of medications you now take, you should also list any experience you have had in treating sinusitis in the past. Such information should include any medications you have taken and what the results were when you took the medication. If you have had any surgery for sinusitis, a nasal operation such as a septoplasty or a rhinoplasty, as well as any other surgery in your face, head, or neck, you should certainly also list for your doctor when the surgery was performed and what the results have been.

ANY PRIOR CT OR MRI SCANS OF YOUR HEAD OR SINUSES

If you have had a prior CT or MRI scan, you should try to obtain the films and bring them with you for the otolaryngologist to review. To make the most accurate diagnosis, the specialist will want to see the actual films, rather than just the report.

A LIFESTYLE DIARY

Because sinusitis may also be affected by certain lifestyle choices, it is also very helpful to the doctor if you bring a diary of your normal activity during a week. Below is a sample.

DATE	ACTIVITY	TIME OF ACTIVITY	LOCATION
3 days a week	swim	1 hour	YMCA indoor pool
1 day a week	bicycle	3 hours	on country roads
in summer	work in flower garden	Varies	in my yard
weekend	go to bar	3 to 4 hours	local restaurant / smoking allowed

As can be seen by this activity chart, this fictitious patient swims in a chlorinated pool, exercises vigorously in an area where crops are grown, works in a flower garden that would be full of pollen, and spends at least three to four hours a week in a place where smoking is allowed. All of these activities could be a cause of sinusitis and would thus be important factors for the doctor to consider.

If you are exposed to some unusual things in the environment, it is important that you list these and discuss them with your physician.

For instance, if you are exposed to chemicals at work, this should be discussed. Similarly, if it appears that allergies may be a factor in your problem, it will be important that you are also tested for any unusual allergens to which you may be exposed.

What Will the Doctor Ask You?

Before the doctor sees you, you will likely be asked to fill out a detailed medical questionnaire. This questionnaire will ask for the following information:

1. Date
2. Identifying data about you (age, sex, race, place of birth, marital status, occupation, and so on)
3. A detailed family history of your blood relatives
4. If you have been referred by another doctor, as well as the names and addresses of that doctor or other doctors who have treated you
5. Present illnesses or complaints you may have (usually this will be in the form of a checklist)
6. Illnesses or complaints you have had in the past (sometimes this is part of the same checklist as your past medical history)
7. A review history asking if you've had problems with any of your other bodily systems, such as urinary tract, lungs, skin, heart, and other organs
8. Surgeries you may have had, particularly surgeries in the head or throat
9. What medications you are now taking; the list you prepared could be used for this
10. Allergies
11. Whether you smoke or drink alcohol and, if so, how much
12. Whether you take any narcotic drugs

13. Whether you have received treatment for mental illness
14. You may also be asked to complete a HIPAA waiver; this allows your doctor to share the medical information with certain specified medical professionals relevant to your medical care

Doctor-Patient Interaction

In most offices, a nurse or assistant will escort you to either the doctor's office or the examining room. A nurse or nurse practitioner may initially review your records with you. The doctor will then review your records and to speak with you about them. This medical interview will allow you to openly discuss your history (past and present) privately with your doctor. This portion of the visit usually includes a review of the forms you filled out, as well as any supporting documents you bring. The doctor will ask many questions and will direct the conversation in a manner that best identifies potential problems.

Most doctors prefer to discuss patient histories in this interview privately with the patient, as we have found by experience that many patients will not disclose detailed personal information in front of family members or friends. If you wish to have a family member or friend present, you should be prepared to answer personal questions with them in the room.

Younger patients still living with parents or very elderly patients often assume that they should have their parents or adult children in the room with them throughout the consultation with the doctor. While this is sometimes desirable, unfortunately, many parents or adult children insist on speaking *for* their children or elderly relatives and it becomes very difficult for the doctor to determine if this information is complete or accurate. If at all possible, unless the child is very young or the elderly person has a memory disorder, it is best if family members wait in the waiting area. Following the examination, the family members can then be asked to join the conversation to discuss further medical tests or medications that may be prescribed.

The Physical Examination

The physical examination performed by an otolaryngologist is typically focused on the head and neck, so you can remain comfortably dressed, although you may be asked to open your collar to allow your neck to be easily felt for any lymph nodes or lumps.

If you suspect you have chronic sinusitis, the otolaryngologist may recommend a nasal endoscopy. This is a simple office procedure in which the physician can examine the patient's nose with a small telescope or endoscope. It allows the doctor to see the nose with much more precision than is possible by just looking into the nose with a light; it usually causes only a little discomfort. However, most physicians will want to spray a decongestant and some local anesthetic into the nose to maximize the benefit of the examination and to ensure minimal discomfort. If local anesthetic is used, it may also numb your throat slightly and, for this reason, it is recommended that you do not eat or drink for an hour or so following the procedure. If you have allergies to any decongestants or anesthetics, or if you are on medications that may interact with nasal decongestants (e.g. the antidepressant medications known as MAOI's), tell your doctor before your nose is sprayed.

Wrap-up Discussion

After the examination, the doctor will discuss with you anything he or she has found, as well as a diagnostic plan and/or any test recommendations. Literature on the subject will be given to you to read. This discussion is usually short, to the point, and directed at a plan. If you wish this portion of the examination to be discussed with a family member or friend, they can be included in the conference. Even at this point, however, some physicians feel that the presence of other people may distract the patient from focusing on the new information that has just been received. This varies from patient to patient, of course. Naturally, this is the time that you may have a number of questions. It is very helpful to the doctor and to your overall care, if you let the doctor know that you have some questions, and then ask them in sequence when he or she is ready for them, rather than interrupting the train of thought while he or she is outlining a treatment plan or filling out a prescription. This will also decrease the potential for errors.

After this portion of the consultation, you will either be sent to the laboratory for blood work, or to a secretary to schedule various tests.

After the evaluation, if a workup is indicated, a long-term plan including a diagnosis and a treatment schedule is initiated. Many sinusitis patients are asked to see their physicians a few times a year, some more frequently, depending on the severity of symptoms. After each office visit with a specialist, the doctor will typically share the current findings with the referring physician, as well as the results of any tests the specialist ordered for you.

After your symptoms are under control, the specialist will advise both you and your referring doctor that his treatment has been completed. At this point, your family doctor will often take over your general care based on the otolaryngologist's recommendations. In more complicated cases, though, you may need to see the specialist on a long-term basis.

Diagnostic Testing and Continued Visits to the Specialist

After an examination, the doctor may suggest that you undergo some diagnostic tests. These tests will be described in the following chapter. If no further tests are necessary, the physician might prescribe a medication for you to take. In any case, a follow-up appointment is usually scheduled in the near future to review your condition.

5

DIAGNOSIS

Including a Review of the Latest Diagnostic Tests

THE SYMPTOMS OF SINUSITIS MAY BE QUITE similar to those of other conditions or diseases, like a cold, influenza, toothache and so on. Thus, in order to treat you effectively, it will first be necessary to make a diagnosis that specifically identifies your condition and that also rules out other causes for your symptoms.

The information-gathering process we discussed in Chapter 4 is the first step in making a diagnosis. As soon as we have all this information, we can move on to the second step, which is an analysis of your symptoms.

Analysis of Your Symptoms

After carefully studying the written information you have provided, the doctor will also want to spend some time talking with you directly. Direct conversation builds on the information gained through the written documents and helps the doctor understand the more intangible and subtle nature of your distress. To begin with, the doctor will probably ask you three questions:

1. What is the quality of your primary complaint? Is it mild, moderate, or severe?

2. What does it feel like? Is it present every day? Every few weeks? On a seasonal basis? On a recurrent basis? (That is, does it come back every week or so throughout the year?)

3. How long does it last? When you have discomfort, does it last for a few hours? A few days? A few weeks?

Direct Observation

After you have answered these questions, your doctor will proceed to the third diagnostic step, conducting an examination to discover what can be determined externally. During this observation, the doctor will probably look at your throat, the inside of your mouth, in your ears, and in your nose. Sometimes a decongestant will be sprayed into your nose, so that the doctor can see what it looks like when the mucosa have shrunk down and the cavity is more visible. Your physician will probably also check for swelling in the lymph nodes in your throat, and may put mild pressure on various points on your face to detect pain caused by pressure in the sinuses. Sometimes the doctor will check your sinuses by placing a light on your skin above and below your eyes. If the sinuses are clear, the light will often shine through the sinuses, lighting up your forehead (frontal sinus) and mouth (maxillary sinus) somewhat like a jack-o'-lantern. This test, which is termed sinus transillumination, is not very accurate because problems or conditions other than inflammation may stop the sinuses from lighting up (for instance, a small sinus). Therefore, most otolaryngologists prefer to rely on a sinus X-ray or C-T scan if they need to confirm their clinical suspicions. However, sinus transillumination in skilled hands can be almost as accurate as an X-ray, is cheaper, and avoids any radiation exposure.

Ruling Out Other Diseases

The fourth diagnostic step is to rule out other diseases as a cause of your symptoms. This is a particularly important step because treatment of diseases, even those with similar symptoms, may be very different in order to be effective. The following are some of the diseases that most commonly share symptoms with sinusitis, and which must be ruled out before a treatment program for sinusitis is prescribed.

THE COMMON COLD. The common cold and sinusitis are interrelated diseases for the simple fact that a cold is often the cause of a sinus infection. Not surprisingly, the symptoms are often the same. As the treatment of sinusitis may be different from the treatment of a cold, however, it is important that a doctor determine which illness you have. A cold is a very common disease both in the United States and around the world. It is estimated that Americans suffer more than a billion colds a year, most of them occurring in children, who may expect to have from 5 to 10 colds each year. Even though colds are very common, there is not yet a cure, perhaps because the same disease can be caused by one of more than 200 kinds of viruses! Most colds in adults are caused by coronaviruses, which also cause diseases in animals and which appear to be at least partially responsible for the newly discovered disease, severe acute respiratory syndrome (SARS). Another culprit is the rhinovirus, of which there are more than 100 known types. Less frequently, colds are caused by adenoviruses, coxsackieviruses, echoviruses, orthomyxoviruses, paramyxoviruses, respiratory syncytial viruses, and enteroviruses. In some cases—perhaps as many as 50 percent of all cases—it is simply not known what caused the sufferer to get a cold.

Although weather was once thought to be the culprit, scientists at the National Institute of Allergy and Infectious Diseases, a division of the National Institutes of Health, now think that being out in the cold (or heat) or, for that matter, what you eat and how much you exercise, are probably unrelated to getting a cold. It is thought, however, that allergies (particularly those that affect the nose and throat), stress, and menstrual cycles may have an effect on whether or not you get a cold. One study, in which more than 200 individuals had colds induced experimentally, it was demonstrated that the volunteer was significantly more likely to develop symptoms if he or she had evidence of stress. The reason more people get colds in the winter is probably more related to the fact that they are indoors and around other people who have colds than anything else they may do.

Cold symptoms typically include a runny nose, obstruction of the nasal passages, sneezing, sore throat, cough, and headache. Some people get a fever with a cold, but a high fever or a fever that lasts for more than a day or two along with these symptoms is usually a symptom of influenza instead.

Although colds are caused by viruses, they can sometimes lead to secondary bacterial infections in the sinuses. In general, if the symptoms are getting worse after 5 to 7 days, or if they are persisting longer than 10 to 12 days, you probably should see your doctor. This would suggest that you may be developing a bacterial infection, or have something other than a cold. It is also wise to see your doctor if the symptoms are particularly severe. Please be aware that only the *symptoms* of a cold can be treated, as there is currently no cure for the disease itself; however, if the cold leads to a bacterial infection in the sinuses, the infection can be treated with antibiotics. A medication under development has been shown in trials to shorten and lessen the symptoms of a cold by blocking the virus. It may be released in the next few years.

INFLUENZA. Although colds are very common, only about 10 to 20 percent of Americans will catch influenza each year. Like a cold, influenza is caused by a virus and is contagious—that is, you get it from contact with another person. Colds, influenza, and sinusitis share some common symptoms such as headache, cough, sore throat, and nasal congestion but influenza symptoms are also likely to include body aches, tiredness, and fever. While there is no cure for influenza, vaccines are now available to prevent it. Vaccines are made from killed viruses, which are changed each year to adapt to the various strains of influenza that appear each year.

Since there are so many different kinds of influenza viruses, the Centers for Disease Control and Prevention (CDC) generally advise vaccinations for people older than age 50, residents of nursing homes, and anyone else who suffers from long-term illnesses. Flu shots are also advisable for children older than 6 months who have chronic heart or lung conditions, such metabolic diseases as diabetes, chronic kidney disease, or a compromised immune system, as with HIV/AIDS. Many doctors recommend that public service employees, for example, police officers and teachers, also get flu shots, since they are exposed to so many people who may have the flu. Of course, now that the vaccines are widely available, anyone who is basically healthy can get a flu shot, if they wish to lessen the chances that they will get the flu. In general, flu shots are safe, although it is possible that some people may have allergic reactions to them. Check with your doctor if you have any questions about whether you or members of your family should get a flu shot.

Three symptoms often ascribed to the flu—nausea, vomiting, and diarrhea—while commonly caused by viruses, are not actually symptoms of influenza. Influenza is a respiratory disease; nausea, vomiting, and diarrhea are symptoms of a disease of the gastrointestinal tract.

ALLERGIES. Allergies that affect the respiratory system can also have the same symptoms as sinusitis—specifically, sneezing, coughing, itchy eyes, and a runny nose. In general with allergies, the nasal discharge is clear and watery, similar to the onset of a cold. Allergies are generally categorized as being either seasonal (occurring at only certain times of the year) or perennial (those that occur year-round). While people may be allergic to just about anything, those with sinusitis-like symptoms are generally allergic to dust, pollen, mites, animal dander, or mold. Although the symptoms of allergies may be similar to those of sinusitis, treatment of allergies is very different from treatment of sinusitis, and what is effective for one disease generally will not work for the other. On the other hand, people who suffer from chronic rhinosinusitis may have nasal allergic reactions that are more pronounced, and there may be significant nasal congestion in response to triggers that they are not normally allergic to, such as smoke, perfumes, and drinking alcohol. If it is unclear to you whether you are suffering from an allergy or sinusitis, you should consult with your doctor to determine the appropriate treatment for your symptoms.

If allergies are suspected of playing a significant part in your problem, your physician may suggest allergy testing. Allergy testing can be performed with either a blood test or with skin pricks. Properly performed and properly interpreted, both types of testing are equally accurate. If you are going to have allergy testing, it is important that you do not take antihistamines for approximately one week prior to the tests, because these can affect the results. However, it is acceptable to continue with any topical steroid treatment because these do not affect the allergy test. It will also be very important that the doctor knows if you are exposed to any unusual allergens (for example, a pet bird or pet rabbit), so that these are included in the testing.

MIGRAINE. Headache is a symptom of acute sinusitis and can be severe. However, it is less common in chronic sinusitis and, in contrast to what we often see in TV advertisements for sinus medications, the headache in chronic sinusitis is usually not as severe; it is more of a feeling of pressure or fullness related to the area of sinus involvement. (See Chapter 2.)

There are many causes for headache, including stress, muscle spasm, neck problems, and temporomandibular joint disorder, to mention just a few. Vascular headaches or migraine headaches are the more common types of recurring headaches. No one knows for sure what causes migraines, but many believe it is a hereditary condition, because approximately 70 percent of those who have migraines have family members who are also migraine sufferers. Additionally, among those who have recurrent migraine, about 75 percent are women. Duration of migraine pain varies from patient to patient as it does for sinusitis sufferers, although migraine pain is usually described as "throbbing" or "pounding," whereas a sinus headache is generally described as a constant, dull pain. While those with sinusitis may experience a headache in several places, migraine sufferers usually find that their pain is located on one side of the head. Headache pain with sinusitis or with migraine can also be aggravated by activity. However, sinusitis sufferers usually find that the pain is worse when they first get up in the morning. Those with migraines may get their headache at any time of the day and any activity or movement, even the slightest one, may bring on pain.

Additionally, those suffering a migraine often experience nausea and vomiting (not usually a symptom of sinusitis), or may find that they have unusual sensitivity to light, sounds, and smells just before a migraine. These are seldom symptoms of sinusitis. Migraine headaches can sometimes be alleviated with dietary changes, and effective migraine medications have been available for a number of years. Consult your doctor if you have frequent recurrent headaches. Unless you have other significant sinus symptoms, it is not likely that sinus disease is the underlying cause of a migraine.

TRIGEMINAL NEURALGIA. Unlike sinusitis, which is a disease caused by bacteria or a malformation of the nose or sinuses, trigeminal neuralgia is a disorder of the nervous system, particularly the nerves in the face. While an acute sinus infection can cause facial pain, the pain caused by trigeminal neuralgia is usually described as much more of an intense, electric shocklike pain in the lips, eyes, nose, scalp, forehead, upper, or lower jaw. Because it is a disorder of the nervous system, antibiotic therapy is ineffective. Trigeminal neuralgia is treated with anticonvulsant drugs or antidepressants. Some patients find relief from this disorder by alternative medicines or acupuncture.

TEMPORAL ARTERITIS. Like trigeminal neuralgia, temporal arteritis may result in symptoms that include pain in the face, pain when chewing, and recurrent severe headaches usually on one side. But temporal arteritis has nothing to do with the sinuses. Rather, it is an inflammation of the temporal artery that runs over the temple in most of the ear. This area is often tender to the touch. Again, antibiotics have no effect on this disorder. It is treated with cortisone or cytotoxic drugs, gammaglobulin, cyclosporins, or plasmapheresis (the removal and reinfusion of blood plasma).

DENTAL AND GUM DISEASE. Because the maxillary sinuses are located near the teeth, what seems like a toothache may be sinusitis. Similarly, what you may at first think is sinusitis may, in fact be an infection in your teeth or gums. Infection in the gums (periodontal disease) occurs in children and young adults, but is most common in adults older than age 35. In fact, it is estimated that up to 75 percent of all American adults have some kind of gum disease. Gum diseases include gingivitis (inflammation of the gums caused by buildup of plaque and food debris) and periodontitis (a more serious disease causing inflammation, loss of bone, bleeding, puffiness, or tooth loss). In addition to pain, symptoms of gum disease include bad breath (halitosis), tenderness, and redness of the gums. Inflammation in a tooth may cause sensitivity to heat, cold, and pressure. These are not usually symptoms of sinusitis.

Fortunately, most gum disease can be cured by good dental hygiene including brushing, flossing, and use of an antibacterial mouthwash. An antibiotic is also sometimes prescribed. If gum disease is allowed to progress, however, surgery is sometimes required. An abscessed tooth will either require removal or a root canal. If a dental infection is not treated, it may spread to the sinuses.

TEMPOROMANDIBULAR DISORDER. Pain in the jaw may indicate a gum disease or sinusitis, but it may also suggest temporomandibular disorder, a group of conditions that affect not the sinuses, gums, or teeth, but the jaw. Included are disorders of the jaw muscles, temporomandibular joints, and nerves. Sometimes referred to as temporomandibular jaw disorder (TMJ), this disorder is sometimes caused by excessive strain on the jaw muscles, clenching the jaw, or chewing gum. It is also more likely to occur if the upper and lower teeth do not meet together correctly. In addition to jaw pain, symptoms may include headache, pain behind the eyes, in the face, shoulder and neck, earache, clicking or popping of the jaw, dizziness, sensitivity of the teeth, and even numbness or tingling sensation in the fingers. The symptoms, while painful or even frightening, are generally not serious. Because this disorder is not an infection, it is generally treated with pain relievers, relaxation techniques, stress management, behavior modification, physical therapy, ice or hot packs, cessation of chewing gum, or, in some cases, surgery. Orthodontic devices, many of which are designed to be used only at night, may also provide significant relief from the symptoms caused by TMJ.

FOREIGN OBJECTS IN THE NOSE, NASAL PASSAGE, OR MOUTH. Children commonly place foreign objects in their nose, and the result can be an interference with the flow of mucus within the sinuses. If it is not noticed, the child may develop an infected, foul-smelling discharge from one side of the nose. Generally, an adult can see the object and remove it when it first happens, although if the object appears to be wedged in and will not come out easily, it is always a good idea to see your doctor so that you do not damage the nose.

Also, if sterile instruments are not used in piercing the nose, lips, or tongue, or if good hygiene is not maintained after a piercing, the area around the object (for example, an earring or a nose ring) may become infected and may spread to the nasal cavities. If any inflammation or redness appears around an area that has been pierced, you should remove the object until the redness or swelling is gone or, better yet, see your doctor who may suggest that you take an antibiotic for your infection.

ENLARGED ADENOIDS. In children, enlarged adenoids may sometimes be mistaken for sinusitis. The adenoids, which lie in the back of
the nose (nasopharynx), are composed of lymphatic tissue. During
childhood, they are more prominent because they help the child to
develop his or her immune system. This enlargement may cause some
nasal obstruction or cause the child to sound "nasal." Occasionally,
however, they may also become inflamed, resulting in discolored nasal
discharge, nasal congestion, and also recurrent ear infections. In this
situation, enlarged and inflamed adenoids may be mistaken for sinusitis. Antibiotics are usually the initial treatment for enlarged adenoids.
(See Chapter 2 for more detail.)

Diagnostic Tests

If the cause of your symptoms is not immediately obvious or does not
respond to treatment, your doctor may ask you to have one or more
diagnostic tests performed.

ENDOSCOPY. An endoscopy is a procedure performed by an otolaryngologist (or nasal and sinus specialist) and is generally performed
in the doctor's office. Prior to the procedure, your nose would usually
be sprayed with a topical nasal vasoconstrictor and an analgesic such
as pontocaine or lidocaine. (The vasoconstrictor shrinks the membranes of the nose that make it easier for the endoscope to pass into
small recesses during the procedure. The analgesic numbs the area,
which usually makes this procedure painless.) After the analgesic and
vasoconstrictor have been applied, the doctor inserts either a rigid or
flexible fiber-optic instrument called an endoscope into the nose.
This instrument has a bright light attached to it, and may also have a
tiny camera attached to a video monitor. Because the endoscope can
magnify images, it allows the doctor to see minute details.

Both flexible and rigid endoscopes have their advantages and
disadvantages in the nose, and which one the doctor uses is very

physician-dependent. The flexible instrument can be fed through the nose and pointed at the openings of different sinus cavities. However, the image is not as clear as with a rigid telescope, and it is very difficult to take cultures and biopsies with a flexible instrument. Otolaryngologists who specialize in nasal diseases are more likely to use a rigid telescope because they provide a clearer view and because you can manipulate instruments alongside them. In this situation, the specialist looks at the different sinus openings by using endoscopes or telescopes with different angles of view.

Nasal endoscopy is often not necessary during an acute sinus infection, but is helpful if the infection is not getting better or if the infections are recurrent or prolonged. This procedure allows the doctor to check for areas of chronic inflammation, malformations of the nose or sinuses, and also for nasal polyps. An endoscopy has the advantage of showing clearly conditions or problems that cannot be seen on a CT scan, as well as enabling culture samples to be taken at the site of the inflammation. It also avoids the radiation involved in a CT scan. A drawback of the endoscope is that it can only see the openings of the sinuses and not the interior of the cavities unless surgery has already been performed.

BACTERIAL CULTURE. At the present time, most sinus cultures are taken directly from the site of inflammation, using a swab or a small suction collector; the doctor performs it while looking through the endoscope. Occasionally, however, it may be necessary to take a sample directly from inside a sinus. This is done by anesthetizing the nose and then passing a long needle into the sinus and withdrawing or washing out a small amount of fluid. Although this type of "sinus tap" procedure provides the most accurate information, it is less common today because similar information can often be obtained using an endoscope, which is a more comfortable procedure.

At the laboratory, the sample obtained by either technique is placed into a sterile petri dish that contains a growth medium. If, after a specific period of time, no growth appears, it can be determined that no bacteria were present in the sample and, thus, no evidence of bacterial infection. Because it takes a day or two for the bacteria to grow, the laboratory technician will often smear a sample of the material onto a slide and stain it (gram stain) to also look directly for the presence of bacteria. This test gives an approximation of the number and type of bacteria present, but does not provide precise information or let the physician know exactly what type of antibiotic to prescribe. As soon as the bacteria have grown in the petri dish, they will be identified accurately and then tested for sensitivity to different types of antibiotics. As more bacteria become resistant to more and more antibiotics, the information obtained in these cultures is becoming vital in choosing the most effective antibiotic. If it is a first or second infection during a year, the bacteria will likely be sensitive to most antibiotics. However, if you have been on multiple courses of antibiotics recently, it is more likely that the bacteria causing your infection will be resistant to some antibiotics and the most effective antibiotic must be chosen carefully. (See Chapters 11 and 12 for details on specific medications used to treat sinusitis.)

COMPUTED TOMOGRAPHY SCAN. Computed Tomography scan (CT scan; previously called CAT scan—computerized axial tomography) is another tool used to diagnose sinusitis. The CT scan was invented by Godfrey Hounsfield in the early 1970s in England and, by 1976, whole-body scanners were available worldwide. A CT scanner is a specialized X-ray machine that, unlike a standard X-ray machine, produces images that are essentially cross-sectional "slices" of the part of your body the doctor wishes to study. The CT scanner was originally designed as a diagnostic device for diseases of the brain, but it is now used for a variety of diagnostic purposes. Modification of the CT scan parameters in order to obtain the best images of the sinuses was originally done by James Zinreich, MD, a colleague, friend, and professor of radiology at Johns Hopkins with whom I

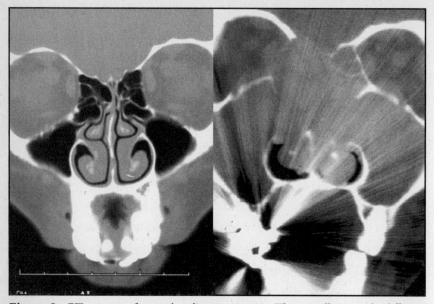

Figure 8. *CT scans are often used to diagnose sinusitis. This scan illustrates the difference between normal sinuses on the left, and inflamed sinuses on the right. The CT scan on the right shows very extensive inflammation of all the sinus and some expansion of the sinuses.*

have worked closely since we first introduced endoscopic techniques into the United States.

During a CT scan, you lie on a bed that is rolled into a long tube. The bed moves slowly forward or backward so the scanner can take the images from different angles. The original CT scanners usually took from four to five or five minutes per image, and the patient was required to lie motionless for long periods of time. During the past 30 years, however, CT scanning technology has improved to the point that an average CT image takes less than a half second, and an entire sinus series can be performed in fewer than 20 seconds. The total length of the test is determined by the number of images required. The scanner does not touch the body and the test is painless. However, it does result in some exposure to radiation and therefore should not be used indiscriminately or too often.

Typically, a CT scan in sinusitis is used to identify the underlying areas of inflammation that may be causing recurrent or persistent episodes of sinusitis. Because the sinuses are affected when a person has a common cold, and the underlying areas will be also masked during or soon after an acute sinus infection, a sinus CT scan for chronic sinusitis should not be performed within two weeks of having a cold, or until an acute sinusitis infection has been treated for several weeks. This will maximize the chances of the CT scan revealing the underlying cause and any areas that may need to be addressed through surgery. Therefore, if you are scheduled for a CT scan and develop a cold or a worsening of your sinus infection, you should let your doctor know. Your scan will probably be postponed unless your physician is concerned about the infection spreading outside the sinus area, in which case a CT scan may be performed without delay.

MAGNETIC RESONANCE IMAGING. Magnetic resonance imaging (MRI) is another diagnostic tool used by doctors to diagnose sinusitis. Early versions of what we now know as MRI were invented in 1946 by Felix Bloch and Edward Purcell, who received the Nobel Prize in Physics in 1952. In 2003, Paul C. Lauterbur of the University of Illinois and Sir Peter Mansfield of the University of Nottingham were also awarded the Nobel Prize for their discoveries concerning improvements in magnetic resonance imaging.

Originally, the invention was known as "nuclear magnetic resonance." It was not used as a medical diagnostic device until the first MRI was performed on a human being in 1977. In that experiment, it took nearly five hours to produce one image. Not widely available as a medical diagnostic tool until the 1980s, however, most large American hospitals now offer MRI testing.

Unlike the CT scan, the MRI uses magnets to produce images. Because no radiation is involved in MRI, there is no radiation exposure risk to the patient and there are usually no side effects. As with a CT scan, the patient lies on a bed that is moved into a large tube.

After receiving direction from the doctor, the technician operating the MRI machine can isolate even very small areas within the body and produce three-dimensional models of that area.

The advantage of MRI over CT is that it differentiates various types of soft tissues. This is very difficult to do with CT. Therefore, MRI is very helpful in detecting tumors, fungal infections, and other problems. However, MRI it is not as good as CT in the diagnosis of routine sinusitis because it does not image bone; the integrity of the bone and any thickening that may occur in the bone as a result of chronic inflammation are important for sinusitis diagnosis. Because MRI involves powerful magnets, it is also not appropriate for patients who have pacemakers or implanted items that are made of steel or other ferromagnetic metal. At the present time, many screws and implants are made of titanium, a non-ferromagnetic metal, and are therefore safe in an MRI scanner. If you have an implant, it is important to know the type of metal that was used in the device; also check with the physician who placed it whether or not an MRI is advisable. People who are very claustrophobic may not good candidates for MRI, because they must remain as motionless as possible, usually for about a half hour, inside a confined space. If you are claustrophobic and need an MRI, there are two alternatives. The best one is for a mild sedative to be prescribed that you can take a couple of hours before the study. The second is to have the MRI performed in an "open magnet"—a machine in which the patient is not completely encased in the device. Unfortunately, open magnets do not provide nearly as clear a picture as a standard MRI and significantly compromise the study's diagnostic accuracy. Additionally, all MRI machines make a lot of noise, similar to hammering, although patients are usually offered earplugs or headphones to muffle the noise. A final drawback is that an MRI is very expensive. If such a test is not covered by your insurance, the cost of the test may be prohibitive.

TRANSILLUMINATION. Transillumination is one of the simplest diagnostic tests. By turning off the room lights and shining a very bright light through the cheek and above the eye, the doctor evaluates how well the light shines through the maxillary and frontal sinuses. If the sinuses are clear, the doctor will see a glow in the mouth or in the cheeks. The advantages of this test are that it is very quick, easy, and completely painless to the patient. The drawback is that it is not very accurate and can suggest a problem when all that is present is just a normal variation in the size of the sinus. If the doctor senses that the problem may be an infection or structural problem within the sinuses, more sophisticated tests may need to be performed.

ULTRASOUND. Although ultrasound has not been used extensively in diagnosing sinusitis, in certain instances, it can be useful. First described in 1942 by Karl Theodore Dussik of Austria, and then in the 1950s by Ian Donald of Scotland, ultrasound is a type of imaging that relies on high-frequency sound waves and their echoes. Ultrasound is similar to the echolocation system used by whales and dolphins to communicate and sonar used in submarines.

Ultrasound works by transmitting high-frequency sound pulses into your body through a probe held by the technician administering the test. The sound waves travel through your body and are reflected back into the probe and transmitted to a computer that calculates the distances from the probe to the tissue or organ the doctor has asked the technician to study.

One advantage of ultrasound is that it can show moving images in "real time" and is now used extensively to study fetuses in the womb without causing any danger to the baby or mother. Ultrasound is also very useful in evaluating the thyroid gland and masses in the abdomen or pelvis. However, it is no longer commonly used for the diagnosis of sinus disease in the United States because the sound waves stop when they hit an air pocket. Therefore, even if you have only a small amount of air in the front of the sinus, the sinus may look normal in an ultrasound image, despite the fact that other parts of the sinus are severely blocked.

X-RAYS. Until the invention of the CT scan and MRI, X-rays were the most common imaging technique used to diagnose acute sinusitis. The X-ray was discovered in Germany in 1895 by Wilhelm Conrad Roentgen, who was awarded the Nobel Prize in 1901 for his discovery. In 1899, the creation of the X-ray tube by C. H. F. Muller, made commercial application of X-rays available and, although they were unaware of the long-term effects of radiation on the human body, doctors were quick to begin using this amazing new diagnostic tool.

Then, as now, X-rays work by focusing radiation into a beam that can pass through most objects, including the human body. The image created by this beam is captured on photographic film placed on the opposite side of the body from the X-ray beam. The film is then developed, and the result is the negative image with which you are probably familiar. The denser the tissue, the more it absorbs X-rays, so dense tissues like bones appear white on the X-ray.

It may be of interest to note that another very early application of X-ray technology was baggage screening at railroad stations. Some of you may also remember that in the 1950s, many shoe stores routinely X-rayed feet to see how well the shoes fit. We now know that prolonged exposure to radiation can be very harmful. Fortunately, in the more than one hundred years since the discovery of X-rays, the technology has greatly improved, the amount of radiation used in a standard X-ray has greatly decreased, and accurate results can now be obtained with little risk to most patients.

X-rays are still sometimes used in diagnosing sinusitis. While X-rays are useful in diagnosing sinusitis in the maxillary or frontal sinuses, they are not useful for seeing problems in the ethmoid or sphenoid sinuses. More than one X-ray is usually needed to provide a true picture of what is going on in the maxillary or frontal sinuses.

X-rays are still sometimes used to determine if symptoms are caused by problems in the jaw or the teeth, however, and they can also show if there is any abnormality in the bone structure of the nose. In general, the information provided by standard (plane film) X-rays in sinus disease is only slightly better than that provided by transillumination. Additionally, X-rays are not useful in diagnosing sinusitis in small children, since their sinus cavities are not completely developed. In general, if the goal is to detect and diagnose sinus disease, it is worth undergoing an MRI or CT scan, despite the fact that CT carries a somewhat higher radiation dose in addition to its higher cost.

6

ACUTE, CHRONIC, AND RECURRENT SINUSITIS

How to Tell What Kind of Sinusitis or Rhinitis You May Have

ORE THAN 90 PERCENT OF AMERICANS will get at least one cold per year, and between 10 and 20 percent will get influenza. With both of these diseases, frequently the sinuses will become inflamed or develop some fluid within them. The inflammation caused by these infections (viral rhinosinusitis) usually spontaneously goes away, and is completely gone in about two weeks. Fortunately, only a very small percentage of people with viral infections end up with a bacterial rhinosinusitis that requires antibiotics.

How do you know whether you have a cold, the flu, or rhinosinusitis? One way is by the symptoms. We've discussed those in detail in Chapter 3. Another way is by the duration of your discomfort. If what you thought was a cold just won't go away, you might well have bacterial rhinosinusitis.

For purposes of treatment, rhinosinusitis is characterized as one of three types: acute, chronic, and recurrent.

Acute Rhinosinusitis

Acute rhinosinusitis is generally defined as rhinosinusitis that is fairly short-lived. Usually, after a diagnosis is made and treatment has begun, discomfort will last only around two weeks. Its onset is also fairly rapid, that is, you can suddenly wake up one day with the symptoms. When acute rhinosinusitis is viral in origin, patients usually recover within five to seven days on their own without medication. If, however, the rhinosinusitis is caused by bacteria, it may persist and slowly worsen, sometimes (although rarely) spreading into the orbital area (eyes) or to the meninges (the membranes that surround the brain and spinal cord). The potential for infection to spread into the orbital area (orbital cellulitis) is significantly greater in infants and small children.

Rhinosinusitis that spreads into the meninges (meningitis) can occur in teenagers and young adults, although it most often develops (about 70 percent of the time) in children younger than age five. Meningitis is a serious disease that can even be fatal—about 10 percent of meningitis patients die. And even though most people survive meningitis, it can leave lasting side effects such as brain damage or loss of sight, hearing, or speech. Both meningitis and orbital cellulitis are medical emergencies, and should be treated immediately. See Chapter 9 for a fuller description of the symptoms of meningitis.

Subacute rhinosinusitis is a low-grade continuation of acute sinusitis and may last more than four weeks, but usually fewer than twelve.

Chronic Rhinosinusitis

Chronic rhinosinusitis is defined as sinusitis that lasts for at least 12 weeks. Sometimes chronic rhinosinusitis is the result of untreated or inadequately treated acute rhinosinusitis. Not surprisingly, by the time the rhinosinusitis becomes chronic, most people will have made at least one or more attempts at medical treatment.

Why some people develop chronic rhinosinusitis is not fully understood, but we think that there are three primary reasons listed below.

1. Environmental factors: These factors may include smoke, air pollution (outside or inside buildings or aircraft with circulating air), viruses, molds, and other allergens in the air.

2. General host factors: These include immune deficiency abnormalities such as HIV/AIDS or cystic fibrosis, asthma, or adverse reaction to aspirin or other non-steroidal anti-inflammatory drugs.

3. Local factors within the nose and sinuses, including nasal polyps, malformation of the nose, damage to the lining of the nose caused by overuse of nose drops and sprays, or nasal cocaine use.

Whereas most people recover completely from an episode of acute rhinosinusitis, chronic rhinosinusitis may persist stubbornly, resisting medical treatment to the point that the only option may be surgery.

In some people, chronic rhinosinusitis may just be a nuisance with some nasal fullness, discharge down the back of the throat, and decrease in the sense of smell. However, in other people, it can become a disorder that impacts their ability to function normally. In these patients, the disease can cause constant discomfort, interfere with sleep, lead to chest infections, and worsen asthma. It is like having a severe cold on a constant basis. It takes little imagination to understand how this can seriously affect a person's ability to function in everyday life.

Interestingly, although severe pain may occur in acute rhinosinusitis, it is very rare in chronic rhinosinusitis. Although an acute rhinosinusitis infection may spread to the area around the eye or the brain, this is also less common when the disease has been present for a significant period of time.

Recurrent Rhinosinusitis

Recurrent rhinosinusitis is defined as repeated incidents of sinusitis that occur over a period of time despite medication and/or surgical procedures. One of the difficulties in diagnosing recurrent rhinosinusitis is determining if the infection is a viral rhinosinusitis (a common cold) or whether it is an acute recurring bacterial rhinosinusitis.

Distinguishing One Kind of Rhinosinusitis from Another

Because rhinosinusitis is such a common disease, most family doctors can usually diagnose acute sinusitis correctly and treat it effectively. But if it becomes recurrent, the patient probably needs to be seen by an otolaryngologist. Generally, a cold will start to improve in about five days, but bacterial rhinosinusitis will typically continue to worsen, often persisting beyond two weeks.

Increasingly discolored nasal discharge is another sign of bacterial rhinosinusitis. However, this symptom is not very reliable in determining what kind of rhinosinusitis may be present because the nasal discharge will also tend to become discolored after several days of a viral infection. If a doctor suspects that a patient may have recurrent rhinosinusitis, diagnostic procedures like those described in Chapter 5 will usually be performed and a course of treatment, possibly involving surgery, medication, and other treatments, may be prescribed.

7

CAUSES OF
SINUSITIS AND RHINITIS

Including Allergy, Asthma, and Other Factors

SINUSITIS IS USUALLY CAUSED BY AN INFECTION from a bacteria, virus, or fungus. In addition, there are many underlying factors that contribute to rhinosinusitis. As mentioned in Chapter 6, it is useful to think of these factors in three different categories:

1. Factors in the environment that predispose an individual to sinusitis.
2. General problems in an individual that may predispose that person to rhinosinusitis.
3. Abnormalities or inflammation in the nose and sinuses that may also predispose a person to rhinosinusitis.

Viral Infections

A virus is a very small, infectious organism, smaller than fungi or bacteria. Viruses live and reproduce by attaching to a cell, releasing DNA or RNA, and taking over the function of that cell. Most viruses can be transmitted from person to person; thus, most viral diseases are contagious.

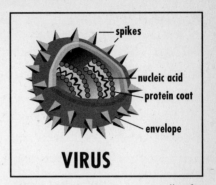

Figure 9. *Viruses are very small infectious organisms that reproduce by attaching to a cell, releasing DNA or RNA, and taking over the function of the cell. Sinusitis can be caused by viruses.*

The body has various mechanisms for defending itself against viruses. The first is the skin. Most viruses cannot get through the skin unless there is an open wound. The mucous membranes in the nose and sinuses are a second, if less effective, barrier to viruses. In fact, one of the most common ways of catching a cold is by touching the nose or the eye after touching someone with a cold or an object on which the virus rests. This is a strong argument for hand washing when around people with colds. The body's immune system is a third barrier. If a virus gets into the body, generally the body launches an attack on the virus (and the cells it may have infected). This attack is carried out by specialized white cells such as lymphocytes (as discussed in Chapter 3).

Vaccines now exist that prevent most people from getting many common viral diseases, particularly childhood diseases such as measles, mumps, and chickenpox. Vaccines also prevent people from contracting various strains of influenza, hepatitis, encephalitis, polio, and smallpox. Unfortunately, no vaccine is yet effective against the common cold. This is particularly unfortunate as colds are the most frequent causes of rhinosinusitis.

Colds are viral infections that often lead to a bout of sinusitis. (See more about colds in Chapter 8.)

Bacterial Infections

Bacteria are single-celled organisms that exist in many forms throughout the environment, including on and inside our bodies. Bacteria are so prevalent in nature that it is estimated that every square centimeter of human skin contains about 100,000 of them.

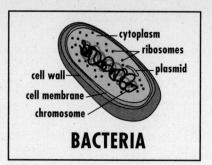

Figure 10. *Bacteria are single-celled organisms that thrive in warm, moist environments such as the sinuses. Bacterial infections are frequently the cause of sinusitis.*

Bacteria are amazingly resilient creatures. They thrive well in warm, moist environments (such as those provided by the human body), but some can even survive in boiling water or subzero conditions. Others can withstand 1,000 times more radiation than humans.

Bacteria were perhaps the earliest forms of life, and are generally credited with helping Earth's atmosphere develop the oxygen that enabled more complex forms of life to evolve. There are many thousands of types of bacteria; however, they normally assume one of three shapes. Rod-shaped bacteria are called bacilli, ball-shaped bacteria are called cocci, and spiral-shaped bacteria are called borrelia.

Although bacteria are responsible for many of the infections we get, they generally do more good than harm. Without bacteria in our intestines, for example, we would be unable to absorb nutrients from our food. It's only when bacteria produce chemicals that are acidic or poisonous to humans that they cause trouble. In addition, when our body's defenses begin to attack the infection, damage to adjacent tissues can also result. Because bacteria can reproduce very quickly—once a minute or so—bacterial infections can become extremely serious if not treated promptly.

STREPTOCOCCUS AND STAPHYLOCOCCUS BACTERIA. The streptococcus pneumonia bacteria most often cause acute rhinosinusitis. In chronic sinusitis, the types of bacteria that are present in the mucus are more varied. Since patients with chronic sinusitis have often taken multiple courses of antibiotics, some of these bacteria may have become resistant to some of the usual antibiotics.

Recently, scientists have begun to look at some toxins produced by relatively common and usually harmless bacteria (staphylococcus coagulase negative), frequently present in the nose, as a potential cause of some of the inflammation seen in chronic rhinosinusitis. Unlike staphylococcus aureus, staphylococcus coagulase negative is found commonly on the body and rarely produces infections. However, it may be that some people may react to a toxin (antigen) that it produces, and that the swelling and inflammation that this reaction produces may be a factor in both chronic rhinosinusitis and nasal polyps. Further research is still ongoing into this so called "superantigen theory" as a factor in chronic rhinosinusitis. It may well turn out to be at least as important as fungi in producing the inflammation associated with this disorder.

The Differences and Interrelationships of Infection and Inflammation

At this point it is helpful to understand the differences and interrelationships of infection and inflammation.

Generally, an infection is defined as the invasion, adhesion, and multiplication of a microorganism in a host. Infections frequently produce pus, a combination of both the organisms that are being killed by the body and the attacking white blood cells that also die in their attempt to control the infection. However, there are also less well-defined infections, for example, those found around the teeth and gums in gingivitis.

The term inflammation is a more general term. Although infections will inflame the tissues, so will many other factors, such as sunburn, constant irritation, or the process of the body reacting to its own tissues as in an autoimmune disorder.

We know that acute bacterial rhinosinusitis is an infection in which pus is frequently found inside one or more of the sinuses. The extent to which chronic rhinosinusitis is an infection, however, is unclear. It appears that chronic rhinosinusitis is actually primarily an inflammation of the tissues, probably from a number of causes, rather than an infection.

Whatever the cause, however, once the tissues are inflamed, the ability of the cilia in the sinuses to move mucus becomes impaired. Mucus then sits on the surface of the lining of the nose and sinuses and, as a result, bacteria begin to grow. This bacterial growth worsens the inflammation. In most cases, however, the bacteria are not the underlying cause of the inflammation.

Although treatment with antibiotics may be helpful in killing the bacteria, unless the underlying inflammation is also treated, the mucus will continue to remain on the surface, and there is the risk that it will, over repeated courses of treatment, cause more infections to occur.

The underlying bone around the sinuses can also become significantly inflamed in rhinosinusitis. It is unclear whether organisms in the bone actually cause the inflammation, or if this is a more generalized type of inflammatory process. In fact it appears to be the latter. However, since bone inflammation is notoriously slow to respond to medical treatment and the inflamed bone undergoes permanent changes, this inflammation does, at least in part, explain why chronic rhinosinusitis takes a long time to respond to medical therapy and is so difficult to treat.

Fungal Infections

To understand how a fungal infection causes rhinosinusitis, it is first important to know a little about fungi. Fungi are living plant-like organisms. They are distinguished from most other plants in that they don't produce chlorophyll, so they must absorb nutrients primarily from dead organic matter. Like bacteria, they can break down many kinds of organic substances and play an indispensable role in the ecology of Earth. We are most familiar with edible fungi such as mushrooms. And many of us are all too familiar with the fungi that grow in damp places in our houses, or seem to thrive in various places in our bodies—primarily dark, moist places like between our toes or, possibly, in our sinuses.

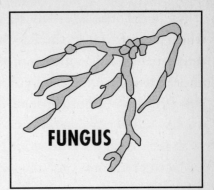

Figure 11. *Fungi are living plantlike organisms that can cause sinus infections. Fungi are particularly a problem for people with auto-immune diseases. Many people are also allergic to fungi.*

Fungi are opportunistic organisms that are especially pervasive when they sense that the body's immune system has been compromised, so fungal infections are especially likely to attack a person who has autoimmune disease or who is ill with any other disease that weakens the immune system. Many people are also allergic to fungi.

Those suffering from true fungal rhinosinusitis infections generally have one of four types of the disease, listed below.

FUNGUS BALL. This type of rhinosinusitis most often occurs in the maxillary sinuses, but can also occur in the sphenoid sinus. In this condition, the fungus lies on the surface of the lining and forms a fungal ball. It is the easiest form of fungal rhinosinusitis to treat and generally goes away once the fungus ball is surgically removed and the associated bacterial inflammation is treated.

ALLERGIC FUNGAL RHINOSINUSITIS. This type of fungal rhinosinusitis affects people who are allergic to fungi commonly found on things all around us and in the air. Those who suffer from allergic fungal rhinosinusitis usually have a healthy immune system, but may have a history of allergies. Typically, patients with fungal rhinosinusitis have thick, sticky, often brown mucus that they can blow out of their nose. Due to its unusual appearance, the mucus they produce is sometimes known as "peanut butter mucus" or "axle grease mucus." As with other rhinosinusitis infections, but particularly fungal infections, those who suffer from this disease may notice a bad odor in their nose. In allergic fungal rhinosinusitis, it is important to open the sinuses surgically, remove all the mucus that is infected with fungi, and then treat the allergic reaction until the sinuses and the inflammation eventually settle down. (More about this in Chapter 13.)

CHRONIC INDOLENT FUNGAL RHINOSINUSITIS. This is also a condition experienced by people who have an otherwise healthy immune system, but in this variation of fungal rhinosinusitis, the fungi actually invades the tissue and then slowly begins to grow. This condition is rare in the United States, but is widespread in some parts of the Middle East and Africa.

FULMINANT FUNGAL RHINOSINUSITIS. Fulminant fungal rhinosinusitis is a form of sinusitis that can lead to aggressive destruction of the sinuses and invasion of the bone structures around the eyeball and brain. This condition is more typical of an immunocompromised patient, particularly a person who has severe, poorly controlled diabetes, HIV/AIDS, or who has received an organ transplant. This is a very serious condition, and immediate treatment, including surgical removal of the tissue containing fungus, is usually indicated.

OTHER TYPES OF CHRONIC RHINOSINUSITIS CAUSED BY FUNGI. Recently, there has been significant interest in fungi as a cause of other types of chronic rhinosinusitis.

Although it does not appear that fungi are the underlying cause of chronic rhinosinusitis, it does appear that, in the same way that some people may react to relatively harmless bacteria in the nose, some also react to the fungi normally found in the nose. In these patients, the fungus acts as a significant irritant, revving up the immune system, and attracting eosinophils (a type of white blood cell) to attack the fungi. These eosinophils, which are also found in people with allergies, then further irritate the mucous membrane in the nose, damaging it and making it more "hyperreactive." In other words, the lining is then more likely to swell in response to a variety of different stimuli. Additionally, it appears that this type of reaction may also be a causative factor in some types of nasal polyps.

Environmental Factors Leading to Sinusitis

Unfortunately, today few of us live in an environment where the air is clean and free of toxins, allergens, and other kinds of pollutants. As a result, many of us are forced to breathe in particles and gasses to which we are allergic, or that can harm the tissues of our nose and sinuses. Seemingly the best we can do is avoid pollutants whenever possible and stay away from things we can control, like smoking or excessive drinking (alcohol tends to dry out the tissues of the throat and irritate its lining). We should also be aware of the symptoms that tell us when we may be developing a cold, influenza, or a case of rhinosinusitis.

The degree to which pollutants and environmental factors bother one person's nose and not another's appears to be, to some extent, genetically influenced. However, in general, pollutants and chemicals also become more bothersome and cause more swelling when the nose is inflamed, essentially setting up a vicious circle in which pollutants cause inflammation and then the inflammation makes the nose more sensitive to further irritation.

AIR POLLUTION. Air pollution is responsible for a long list of respiratory problems, including rhinosinusitis. The mucus created in the nose and sinuses is designed to capture the harmful particles we breathe in and send them to the stomach, where they are killed by stomach acid. Sometimes, however, the air is so saturated with harmful particles that it causes inflammation and swelling of the lining of the nose. This swelling impairs the ability of the cilia to sweep the particles away, and the inflammation then worsens. As a result, the sinuses may become clogged and obstructed and the mucus that is unable to drain becomes infected. Meanwhile, the harmful particles that remain in the nose, sinuses, and throat can irritate the linings of these airways or cause actual damage to them.

SMOKING. Smoking is a bad idea for anyone, since the risks to the health of the respiratory system are so severe. However, smoking is a particularly bad idea for people prone to rhinosinusitis. As we discussed in Chapter 1, the sinuses and nose are lined with tiny hairs (cilia) that propel the mucus along at the correct pace so that the sinuses remain clear and toxins and pollutants are eliminated in a timely manner. Cigarette smoke slows the sweeping action of the cilia and eventually damages them, thereby causing the mucus to accumulate in the sinuses. Because the mucus is not moving as it's supposed to, it also thickens, a situation that causes sinus blockage and a runny nose. Thickened mucus moving down the throat is one reason that smokers develop a chronic cough.

Surgery that helps most people can do more harm to smokers than good. During sinus surgery, small areas of bone are exposed. If someone smokes in the first six weeks or so after surgery, before this exposed bone has regrown the covering, severe scarring may occur, and the sinuses can close even more severely than they did prior to surgery. For this reason, unless it is an emergency, surgery is not recommended for patients who have not yet stopped smoking.

Although secondhand smoke does not pose as serious a problem, it still has some affect on nonsmokers, because those around people who are smoking cannot help but breathe in at least some smoke.

ALLERGIES. Many different types of allergies are thought to be related to rhinosinusitis. (See more about allergies in Chapter 8.)

CLIMATE. For many people, climate appears to play a significant role in rhinosinusitis symptoms. Because fungi thrive in warm, wet conditions, hot, humid climates are often a problem for those who are allergic to molds. Other rhinosinusitis sufferers find that they experience more problems in a low humidity climate. Although there is little doubt that climate can play a role in developing rhinosinusitis, in some cases symptoms that patients attribute to climate may, instead, be the result of air pollution or allergens.

SICK-BUILDING SYNDROME. The so-called sick-building syndrome may also contribute to the incidence of sinusitis in some people. According to the U.S. Environmental Protection Agency, this condition is one in which people who visit, live, or work in a particular structure experience symptoms—although no specific illness or cause can be identified. These symptoms include headache, irritation of the eyes, nose, or throat, dry cough, dry or itchy skin, dizziness, nausea, fatigue, and sensitivity to odors. Nasal congestion may also occur, and it appears that this exposure may trigger chronic rhinosinusitis in individuals who have a predisposition toward sinus problems.

Sometimes it is impossible to identify the exact cause of these symptoms. In other incidences the source of the problem is found to be inadequate ventilation or chemical contamination from materials or substances found inside the building, such as carpeting, chemicals, or cleaning products. In other cases, the cause may be biological contamination from molds, bacteria, pollen, and viruses. In yet other cases the cause may be from "outside" sources, such as air pollution, auto exhaust, or poorly vented plumbing. Often, the cause of symptoms may result from several of these factors occurring simultaneously. Whatever the cause, sick-building syndrome usually occurs because air inside the building is recirculated without sufficient addition of fresh air or proper air cleaning within the heating, air-conditioning, or ventilation systems.

Fortunately, one of the major causes of sick building syndrome—the recirculation of cigarette smoke—is no longer a problem, since few buildings now allow smoking.

COCAINE USE. The majority of cocaine users sniff or snort it through the nose. Not surprisingly, with repeated use, this powerful drug can have significant negative effects on the nose and sinuses, in addition to causing frequent nosebleeds and hoarseness. Over time, the mucous membranes on the septum can dry out and crust and, eventually, the septum can become perforated. When this happens, the user may experience a whistling sound when breathing, a condition often known on the street as "coke nose." Many cocaine users treat their condition with over-the-counter nasal decongestants that, unfortunately, only add to the problem by narrowing the blood vessels and causing more drying out. In the long run, severe and very difficult to treat inflammation can occur with marked nasal congestion and obstruction.

Factors in the Body that May Predispose People to Rhinosinusitis

HEREDITY. Heredity is also thought to play a role in predisposing a person to rhinosinusitis. Sometimes the effects of heredity are easy to see, such as when rhinosinusitis occurs in conjunction with a known inherited disease such as cystic fibrosis. However, the effects of heredity are often much more subtle, so that only one family member may have mild rhinosinusitis or asthma and others may have no problems at all. Yet another family member may have severe rhinosinusitis, asthma, and nasal polyps. A predisposition to allergies also appears to be inherited. In many cases, therefore, it appears that heredity provides a predisposition toward chronic rhinosinusitis, asthma, and allergies, with environmental and other factors also playing significant roles.

Some diseases associated with chronic rhinosinusitis are clearly inherited. One hereditary disease, known as Kartagener's Syndrome, is a condition in which all of the organs are on the "wrong side" of the body (for instance, the heart is on the right side of the chest instead of the left). Kartagener's syndrome is also associated with absent cilia. This means that, in these people, the mucus cannot be moved out of the sinuses or out of the middle ears. As a result, they usually suffer from recurrent pneumonias, fluid in the ears, and chronic rhinosinusitis beginning when they are infants. They may also experience poor sinus development (for example, absent frontal sinuses). Although full-blown Kartagener's syndrome is usually identified early in life (usually when the first chest X-ray is performed), other, less severe inherited abnormalities of the cilia can be more subtle and may not be discovered until reaching adulthood.

CYSTIC FIBROSIS. Cystic fibrosis (CF), the most common fatal genetic disease in the United States, is a chronic, progressive disease of the body's mucus-producing glands. The disease causes the body to produce thick, sticky mucus that clogs the lungs and blocks the pancreas, keeping the digestive enzymes from reaching the intestines. Until recently, people with CF seldom lived beyond childhood. However, with better medical management, people with CF now often live well into adulthood and can participate in most normal lifetime activities. Additionally, now that genetic testing for the disease is available, it has been found that some people with this disorder only have chronic rhinosinusitis, without other significant manifestations of the disease. Studies are now underway to see if the presence of alterations in a gene known as CFTR might also play a role in a wider group of people with chronic rhinosinusitis, but who do not have any history to suggest CF. (More about this in Chapter 17.)

IMMUNE SYSTEM DEFICIENCIES. Some immune system deficiencies are inherited. David Vetter, the famous "bubble boy," had such a serious deficiency that he was forced to live in an isolated environment that protected him from direct contact with virtually everyone and everything until his death at age 12.

Most inherited immune system deficiencies usually become apparent in infancy, with symptoms including recurrent episodes of chest infections, diarrhea, and ear infections. More subtle inherited problems with the immune system may not be identified until adult life. Chronic rhinosinusitis may be one of the frequent symptoms, although a tendency to other infections is also usually present.

HIV is an example of an immune deficiency that is acquired. Many people with HIV develop chronic rhinosinusitis, although it is not yet known exactly why. One theory is that people with HIV, whose autoimmune systems are compromised, are particularly susceptible to bacterial infections of any kind. Another theory is that people with HIV generally develop more allergies than people who do not have the virus. The susceptibility of HIV-positive individuals to rhinosinusitis is, of course, compounded if they are smokers or users of cocaine.

ASTHMA. Asthma is a condition that is characterized by intermittent airway constriction, and is closely related to rhinosinusitis. The increased airway reactivity present in asthma is similar to the increased reactivity of the nasal mucous membranes in chronic rhinosinusitis. Indeed, it has been suggested that chronic rhinosinusitis be called "asthma of the nose" because of the close relationship between the two disorders. (See more about asthma in Chapter 8.)

ASPIRIN ALLERGY. As we'll discuss in Chapter 8, there is a direct correlation between aspirin allergy, asthma, and rhinosinusitis. For example, nearly one-third of people who are allergic to aspirin also have nasal polyps. Even if a severe, life-threatening allergy to aspirin is not present, many people with asthma and nasal polyps will also demonstrate mild evidence of aspirin allergy if carefully tested. Although some people with this disorder (ASA Triad, or Samter's Triad) develop the aspirin allergy first, others may initially experience either asthma or nasal polyps, and the aspirin allergy may not become noticeable until later.

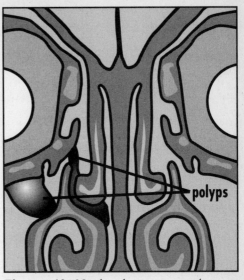

Figure 12. *Nasal polyps are smooth, pear-shaped, semi-transparent growths inside the nose that can sometimes block the airways, causing mucus to back up and become infected.*

HORMONAL IMBALANCES. Unless they are pregnant, women have no greater risk of developing rhinosinusitis than men. However, the hormones released during pregnancy, which are designed to thicken the uterus, also seem to thicken nasal passages resulting in nasal congestion. (More about this in Chapter 16.)

MEDICATION SIDE EFFECTS. Some medications, such as some of those used to treat high blood pressure and depression, may cause rhinosinusitis by creating nasal congestion. Even some of the medications that are used to treat asthma and allergies could potentially cause rhinosinusitis. We will discuss drugs and their side effects in Chapter 11.

Local Factors Around the Nose and Sinuses Predisposing People to Sinusitis

NASAL POLYPS. Nasal polyps are smooth, pear-shaped semitransparent growths inside the nose. Unlike polyps in the bowel, the common polyps found in the nose are not precancerous. They are merely a manifestation of chronic inflammation in the area and are most

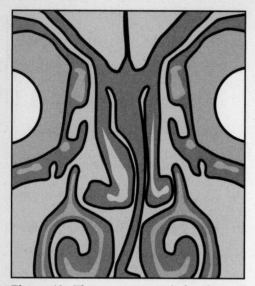

Figure 13. *The septum, composed of cartilage and bone, divides the nose into two nostrils. Most people have a slight deviation in the septum but, if the deviation is severe enough, it can cause nasal obstruction.*

common in middle-aged men. Although only about 2 percent of Americans have nasal polyps, for those who do, these polyps can become a major cause of symptoms of rhinosinusitis because they block the airways, causing mucus to back up and become infected.

There is also a correlation between aspirin allergy, nasal polyps, and asthma (see aspirin allergy above), but by no means will all patients with nasal polyps also have asthma. There is also an association with fungal rhinosinusitis, since the majority of people who have allergic fungal sinusitis have nasal polyps as well.

Nasal polyps may also interfere with the sense of smell, block the nose, and cause it to run. They can also lead to sleep disturbance and be associated with a general feeling of malaise. However, because they typically develop very slowly, the symptoms that the polyps are causing may not be fully recognized by the patient until the problem is corrected. Nasal polyps can be treated medically in some patients, or removed by surgery when they do not respond to medical treatment. (See Chapter 13.) However, surgery does not take away the underlying tendency to grow polyps and, typically, they will regrow if post-operative medical treatment is not also undertaken.

NASAL SEPTAL DEVIATION AND SEPTAL BONE SPUR. The septum is a structure composed of cartilage and bone that divides the nose into two nostrils. Ideally, the septum would divide the nose into two equal nostrils but, more often than not, the nostrils are not equal. In fact, in almost 80 percent of the United States population, the septum deviates in some way. Many people are born with a deviated septum and others end up with this condition as a result of an injury such as a broken nose.

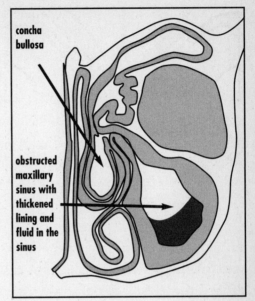

For most people, a slight deviation produces few problems but, for others, the deviation is severe enough to cause nasal obstruction. It can be surgically repaired by a procedure called a septoplasty. (See Chapter 13.)

Figure 14. *Concha Bullosa is an enlargement or ballooning of the middle turbinates, the small bony structures which protrude into the nose.*

A nasal septal deviation may also impair the ability of the sinuses to clear mucus, either by compressing the sinus openings, or by redirecting the nasal airflow in such a way that it dries the mucus. Sometimes, particularly if there has been a prior injury to the nose, the septum may form a bone spur that can pass right up into the area of the middle meatus (where most of the sinuses drain). A septal deformity is therefore a potential cause of chronic rhinosinusitis.

CONCHA BULLOSA. Concha bullosa is an enlarging or ballooning of the middle turbinates, the small, bony structures covered by mucous membranes, which protrude into the nose. As we discussed in Chapter 2, the purpose of these turbinates is to help warm, humidify, and cleanse the air that is breathed in through the nose. Occasionally, however, an ethmoid air cell can grow into the middle turbinate, enlarging it (sometimes massively), leading to obstruction of the adjacent sinus openings, which causes mucus to back up and become infected.

Other forms of enlarged turbinates typically result from allergies or from some early chronic sinusitis and, if they become symptomatic, are best treated by managing the underlying problem rather than by surgery. As discussed in Chapter 2, the turbinates are important baffles for the nasal air passages and should be maintained unless they are irrevocably diseased. However, enlarged turbinates can cause headaches and sleep disorders such as snoring and sleep apnea. (See Chapter 13.)

COSMETIC SURGERY. Cosmetic, or plastic, surgery is generally thought of as surgery designed only to change or enhance an individual, from an aesthetic standpoint. It is possible that some cosmetic surgery, particularly rhinoplasty (surgery of the nose), can interfere with breathing and thus cause rhinosinusitis, particularly in someone who already has other predisposing factors toward chronic rhinosinusitis. In most cases, however, cosmetic surgery not only improves the facial features (at least, in the opinion of the person having the surgery), but may also improve the ability to breathe normally.

INJURY. The nose and sinus cavities are specifically designed to move air and mucus through specific pathways in a particular direction. When injury to the face, such as a facial fracture, alters this pathway in any way, the flow of mucus is sure to be affected and the opportunity for sinusitis occurs. Additionally, even if the sinus does not become infected, if there is blockage of the sinus drainage, a cyst (mucocele) may slowly develop, which might only start to cause symptoms many years later when it has grown much larger. Following an injury to the face, surgery may be required to restore the airways to as close as possible to their original position, as well as to restore any cosmetic deformity. (See Chapter 13.) When surgery is not necessary, medications may be considered to try to ensure that the sinuses continue to drain. (See Chapter 11.)

NASAL AND SINUS TUMORS. Although nasal polyps are not tumors, tumors can sometimes grow in the nose and sinuses, blocking both the nose and sinuses and leading to a secondary sinusitis. The most common tumors in the nose are benign, although cancer can occasionally occur. Typically, they cause obstruction on one side of the nose that gets progressively worse with time. Bleeding may also occur. As the tumors begin to obstruct one or more of the sinuses, repeated episodes of sinusitis may occur.

The most common tumor in the nose is a benign tumor called an inverted papilloma. It is associated with the same group of viruses that cause warts (papilloma viruses) as well as with chronic sinusitis. On initial examination, these tumors can sometimes be mistaken for a nasal polyps, but they are usually solitary and can be diagnosed with certainty by biopsy, something that can be performed in the doctor's office. Although they are benign, they do need to be removed. If not, they will become difficult to remove, and begin to press on the eye or the brain, as well as to destroy the normal nasal structures. They can also occasionally become malignant. Tumors can usually be removed with by endoscopy, without the need for external incisions.

Another, less common, benign tumor occurs only in adolescent males. It is called a juvenile angiofibroma, and is frequently accompanied by recurrent nose bleeds and nasal obstruction. It is important that this tumor be completely removed.

Cancer starting in the nose or sinuses is rare, but can, in some cases, precipitate sinusitis. It is more common in carpenters who work with hard woods and are exposed to their dust. It is also more common in old age.

ADENOIDS. Enlarged adenoids cause one of the most common problems that occur in children and may predispose a child toward either chronic rhinosinusitis or fluid in the ear (serous otitis media). Children who have enlarged adenoids may have trouble sleeping, or may eventually develop dental deformities from breathing primarily through the mouth. In most people, the adenoids shrink on their own and essentially disappear by adulthood. In children, if they remain chronically swollen, they may need to be surgically removed. (See Chapter 13.) Removal of the adenoids is often undertaken as a first procedure in children with chronic rhinosinusitis that does not respond to medical management. It is a relatively benign procedure that may allow the sinuses to settle down.

PROBLEMS IN THE TEETH. Because the upper molars are located near the maxillary sinuses, a tooth infection, which is likely to be a bacterial infection, can spread to the sinus cavities. Such infections usually start in the maxillary sinuses, but can also spread to other areas, too.

Dental implants have become increasingly popular among people who lose their teeth later in life. However, if the bone above the teeth is thin, it may need to be reinforced with a bone graft (sinus lift procedure) before the implants can be placed. This operation can occasionally result in a severe rhinosinusitis complicated by infection of the bone grafts.

SWIMMING AND DIVING. Swimming and diving in polluted water is certainly a health risk for anyone, but for those who suffer from rhinosinusitis, swimming even in chlorinated water can often pose a risk. Some people with reactive nasal mucus membranes and a predisposition toward rhinosinusitis may significantly react to the chlorine in the water, creating both inflammation within the nose (rhinitis) and sinusitis. Diving can also be a problem for people with rhinosinusitis since the change in air pressure may provoke a sinus attack. Ironically, in people with chronic rhinosinusitis, scuba diving, if it does not cause pain, can actually be beneficial, since the change in pressure and salt water may help to drain congested sinus cavities.

AIRPLANE FLIGHT. Many people with a propensity toward rhinosinusitis complain that infections frequently begin following flying. The reason would appear to be a combination of factors. One is the fact that people in an airplane are in close proximity to one another and, because the air is being recirculated, there is a greater likelihood of catching a viral infection. Additionally, the dry air and the pressure changes associated with airplane descent may increase the risk of a bacterial rhinosinusitis.

EXCESSIVE NOSE BLOWING. The mucus in our nose and sinuses only has two places to go, down the throat or out through the nose. Generally, we have little choice as to which way the mucus goes. Occasionally, however, some people will become obsessive about blowing their noses. The results can be harmful rather than helpful, particularly if the nose is blown incorrectly (the nose should be blown one nostril at a time). The nose is intended to be coated with mucus, which not only traps harmful particles from the air, but also lubricates the nose to protect its tissues. Therefore, excess nose blowing can both strip the nose of mucus and make the lining overly dry. Excessive nose blowing can also force mucus that has become contaminated with bacteria into the sinuses, which are normally sterile areas. As a result, people who blow their noses too often may increase their risk of developing a significant bacterial rhinosinusitis.

FOREIGN OBJECTS PLACED IN THE NOSE. Although some adults have been known to occasionally place foreign objects in the nose, children frequently shove food, toys, and other objects into their noses (as well as mouth and ears). Although such objects can generally be removed by observant parents, if the object seems difficult to remove, it is generally a good idea to seek the assistance of a health professional. Persistent foul-smelling nasal drainage from one side of the nose is often a symptom of an object lodged in the nose.

HEARTBURN AND GASTROESOPHAGEAL REFLUX DISEASE. Gastroesophageal reflux disease (GERD) occurs when the acid in the stomach is refluxed back up the esophagus and sometimes up into the pharynx and mouth. In some cases, but not all, this creates heartburn.

Not only does the acid damage the esophagus, it may also cause chronic hoarseness (laryngitis). Reflux is most likely to occur at night. Although the exact relationship is still unknown, there does appear to be a link between GERD and asthma, and there is some suggestion that it could also be a factor in the development of both rhinitis and rhinosinusitis in some people.

8

OTHER RESPIRATORY CONDITIONS AND ALLERGIES

How Other Conditions May Contribute to Sinusitis

Allergies

Today, it is estimated that more than 40 million Americans suffer from allergies. And that number is growing, probably in large part as a result of more pollutants and toxins entering the air we breathe.

Simply put, allergies are a hypersensitivity or reaction of the immune system to allergens (matter that causes allergic reactions) such as pollen, food, or drugs that, in most people, would not produce the same reaction. More specifically, in people with allergies, the body's immune system overresponds to specific, noninfectious things like pollen, pet dander, tobacco smoke, and a long list of other so-called "triggers." The antibodies in the blood, mostly immunoglobin E (IgE), attach to mast cells (cells that release histamine) in the lungs,

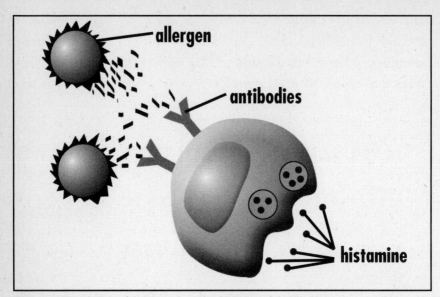

Figure 15. *An allergy is a hypersensitivity, or reaction of the immune system, to allergens like pollen, food, or drugs that in most people would not result in the same symptoms. When an allergic reaction occurs, the body releases histamine that dilates the blood vessels and can result in swollen membranes in the nose, itchy eyes, sneezing, nasal stuffiness, nasal congestion, and drainage.*

skin, and mucous membranes, causing histamine to be released. When this happens, the histamine dilates the blood vessels, and the result is a skin rash or swollen membranes in the nose. Other symptoms include itchy eyes, sneezing, nasal stuffiness, nasal congestion, sinus drainage, and headache.

Most people simply endure allergy symptoms or use one of the many over-the-counter medications now available. If the specific source of the allergy can be identified, either avoidance of the allergen or, in some cases, immunotherapy (allergy shots) may help.

Although it is possible for people to be allergic to just about anything, the most common causes are identified below.

MITES. Mites are microscopic creatures, members of the biological class Arachnid which, along with ticks, are known as acari. Because they constitute the second most diverse group of animals in the world (there are more than 48,000 different species of acari), they exist in virtually every ecosystem on the planet, from our cleanest homes to garbage dumps, and from the Arctic to the midst of geothermal springs. It is now believed that it is the excretion of these tiny creatures that causes an allergic reaction in some people, so even dead mites can cause problems for susceptible humans.

ANIMALS. Many people are allergic to domestic animals. While it might be assumed that the most common allergies are to fur or feathers, it is generally the allergens in the saliva, dander (flaking skin), or urine that cause an allergic reaction in humans. Of all pet allergies, those caused by cats are perhaps the most common; the dander and other allergens can remain in a house for many years after the cat is no longer there.

POLLEN. Many plants reproduce by creating microscopic particles that are transferred from plant to plant by air, animals, or insects. While allergy to pollen is commonly referred to as hay fever, more people are probably allergic to tree pollen, flower pollen, or the pollens of grasses other than hay. Hay fever is also sometimes referred to as seasonal allergic rhinitis.

INSECTS. Insects, particularly insect stings, are another common allergy. While many insects sting, Hymenoptera (bees, yellow jackets, hornets, and wasps) generally produce the worst symptoms. In fact, some people are so allergic to the bites of these insects that death may occur within minutes of a sting.

DRUGS. Almost any drug can cause a reaction, which is why every medication comes with a long list of possible side effects printed on the package insert. However, most drug reactions are not truly allergies. Generally, drug allergies are mild and include headache, upset stomach, diarrhea, or a skin rash. On occasion, however, drug allergies can be severe, causing anaphylaxis, an unusual or exaggerated reaction to a foreign particle or substance that may cause itching and swelling or, in rare cases, difficulty breathing, convulsions, shock, coma, and even death. One of the drug allergies with a specific relationship to both rhinosinusitis and asthma is an allergy to aspirin and other similar nonsteroidal analgesics. Patients who develop this allergy frequently also develop both severe asthma and polyps in the nose and sinuses.

FOOD. Although any adverse reaction to food is often called a food allergy, strictly speaking, not all such reactions are allergies—only those that involve the body's immune system. Other adverse reactions to food are more accurately described as food intolerances, that is, the inability of the body to properly digest them. Common food intolerances include lactose or gliadin, main components of milk and milk products, and grains.

A true allergic reaction to foods involves a stimulation of the immune system, usually resulting in the release of histamine. In particularly sensitive people, a food allergy can result in anaphylaxis, and death may result if immediate medical care is not received. More common symptoms of food allergies include hives, skin rashes, vomiting, diarrhea, and, as we discussed in Chapter 3, a runny nose or swelling of the throat, lips, or tongue.

The foods people are most generally allergic to include shellfish, milk, wheat, nuts, and eggs, although it is certainly possible to be allergic to just about any food.

The Common Cold

As its name suggests, the common cold is the most frequently experienced illness in the world. According to the American Academy of Family Physicians, at least 90 percent of the U.S. population will get at least one cold a year and children, particularly young children, may have as many as a dozen. As we discussed in more detail in

Chapter 3, colds typically involve a runny nose, sinus congestion, sneezing, a sore throat, fever, cough, and mild body aches and last for a week or so.

One of the major misconceptions about a cold is that it is a bacterial infection and thus is helped by antibiotics. In reality, a cold is a viral infection and, as yet, there is no cure. Over-the-counter medications can often lessen the symptoms, but the cold itself will usually run its course no matter what you do. There is also no vaccine to prevent colds. Your best protection is to lead a healthy lifestyle, avoid other people who have colds, and wash your hands often, as viruses are often spread by direct contact with people who have colds.

INFLUENZA. Although it is sometimes difficult to tell whether you have a cold or the flu when you are first coming down with an illness, there are significant differences between the two diseases. The main difference is that they are caused by different viruses. Colds are caused by up to 15 different viruses including the rhinovirus. Influenza is caused by one of the many strains of the influenza virus. Colds and flu share such symptoms as fever, muscle aches, fatigue, and sometimes runny nose, but these symptoms are generally more severe with the flu, and flu sufferers may also experience vomiting, diarrhea, and fatigue lasting several weeks.

While it is possible to be miserable with a cold, most people recover. The flu, however, can be a killer. During 1918 and 1919, more than 20 million people worldwide died of influenza, making it the single worst epidemic in world history.

The Centers for Disease Control estimate that from 10 to 20 percent of Americans will get the flu each year. Most will recover in one to two weeks, but many will develop life-threatening complications such as pneumonia, and approximately 36,000 people will die as a result each year.

One problem with the flu is that it is highly contagious and spread by coughs, sneezes, or touching a person who has it.

Fortunately, there are now several vaccines that can protect people from this disease but, because there are many strains of the disease caused by different viruses, most people need to get a yearly flu vaccination.

Severe Acute Respiratory Syndrome

Sometimes other types of respiratory diseases suddenly occur in the human population without warning. In November 2002, a mysterious pneumonia-like disease known as severe acute respiratory syndrome (SARS) was diagnosed in the Guangdong province of China and quickly spread worldwide, primarily through contact with people who had traveled from China to other countries. Symptoms of SARS include headache, muscular stiffness, loss of appetite, malaise, confusion, rash, and diarrhea. The virus that causes SARS is a member of the Corona family of viruses that includes the viruses that generally cause colds.

Rhinitis and Rhinosinusitis

Rhinitis is an inflammation of the nose. However, because the sinuses are usually also inflamed when the nose is inflamed and vice versa, the term rhinosinusitis is often being used as a term to cover both what used to be considered rhinitis and what used to be considered sinusitis. There are a number of different types of rhinitis, including infectious (basically, a cold), seasonal allergic, perennial allergic, drug-induced, and rhinitis of pregnancy. Another term, vasomotor rhinitis, was frequently used to describe many other forms of rhinitis that were not related to allergies. However, lately it has been recognized that this form of rhinitis in particular probably arises as a result of low-grade sinusitis.

Seasonal allergic rhinitis occurs when the sufferer is allergic to something in the atmosphere like pollen, mold, or one of the other triggers discussed earlier in this chapter. Most people with seasonal allergic rhinitis experience the discomfort of this disease in the spring or late summer when plants are releasing pollen. Although seasonal allergic rhinitis is often referred to as hay fever, as we mentioned earlier, hay is seldom the culprit. More likely it is ragweed, tree, or other types of plant pollen.

Perennial allergic rhinitis may have the same symptoms as seasonal allergic rhinitis, but it usually occurs throughout the year, rather than at a specific time. This disease results from an allergy to one or more of the chemicals or substances mentioned earlier in this chapter.

Although allergic rhinitis is not caused by bacteria, according to the American Academy of Otolaryngology, such bacteria as staphlococcus aureus are often found in the nasal passages of people with perennial allergic rhinitis. This suggests that this type of allergy could lead to higher bacterial levels existing on a regular basis in the nose and sinuses in people with a propensity to allergies.

Rhinitis of pregnancy is caused by hormonal changes and swelling of the turbinates within the nose. It tends to worsen later in the pregnancy but typically disappears after the pregnancy has ended.

Drug-induced rhinitis can occur as the result of a number of medications including some of the medications used to combat high blood pressure or treat depression. However, one of the most common causes is the overuse of topical nasal decongestants (rhinitis medicamentosa). A severe form of drug-induced rhinitis can also be caused by sniffing or snorting cocaine into the nose. Chronic nasal cocaine use can result in bleeding, structural changes to the nose, and a perforation through the nasal septum (septal perforation).

Vasomotor rhinitis was the term used to describe the condition people have when they have a stuffy nose, but don't seem to have specific allergies or a cold. However, we now have better ways to visualize the sinuses, either by using CT scans or by looking into the nose with fiber-optic endoscopes or telescopes. We now know that many of these patients also have some degree of sinusitis that appears to make their nose more reactive (nasal hyperreactivity) to a large number of factors, including changes in climate, perfumes, cigarette smoke, viruses (for instance, the common cold), emotional stress, or reaction to medications. At present, it is recognized that this type of increased nasal reactivity is also closely related to asthma; indeed the term "asthma of the nose" has been suggested because of this close relationship.

Asthma

Asthma is a disorder characterized by intermittent airway constriction and can also be considered a hyperreactivity of the lower airway. Like rhinosinusitis, the incidence of asthma has increased dramatically in recent years. Some researchers have speculated that this may be due, at least in part, to an increase in the incidence of pollution but there is no firm evidence yet to support this theory.

There is a close relationship between asthma and chronic sinusitis. In fact, as many as 75 percent of patients with asthma also report symptoms of sinusitis. There is no supported evidence to suggest that rhinosinusitis causes asthma. However, it is clear that, in asthmatic people, the asthma typically becomes significantly worse and more bothersome when their sinuses are inflamed. Similarly, people with both disorders typically experience a significant improvement in their asthma symptoms when their sinuses are treated, either medically or with surgery.

Although it is still unclear exactly what causes asthma, the result is a spasm in the smooth muscles of the lung, inflammation of the tissues lining the airways, and flow of excess mucus into the airways, causing the sufferer to gasp and wheeze while attempting to breathe.

Asthma was traditionally divided into two types, extrinsic and intrinsic asthma. Extrinsic asthma, which is accompanied by identifiable allergies, is now more commonly referred to as allergic, or atopic, asthma. (Atopy is the genetic tendency to have a specific allergic reaction.) Intrinsic asthma, which is not accompanied by identifiable allergies, encompasses exercise-induced and occupational asthma.

Occupational asthma is found primarily among people who work around chemicals, and more than 200 substances—including flour, sawdust, and formaldehyde—have been found to bring on an attack in those who are sensitive to them.

Up to 90 percent of asthmatic people experience exercise-induced asthma. Whereas in the past, individuals with asthma were discouraged from athletic activity, thanks to some of the newer medications, most people with asthma can now exercise safely.

Asthma frequently becomes worse for a period of time following a common cold, or with an episode of bacterial sinusitis or the onset of postnasal drip. Asthma may also be caused by GERD, especially at night.

The association of asthma, rhinosinusitis with polyps in the nose, and allergy or sensitivity to aspirin (acetylsalicylic acid, or ASA) and nonsteroidal anti-inflammatory medications (NSAIDs) deserves some discussion. NSAIDs include ibuprofen (Motrin®, Advil®, Motrin IB®), naproxen (Naprosyn®, Aleve®), and nabumetone (Relafen®). This disorder is sometimes called either Samter's Triad (after one of the first people to describe the association) or aspirin (ASA) triad. People with Samter's Triad asthma may experience symptoms that can include a gastric upset, a severe asthma reaction, and even a life-threatening allergic reaction, when they ingest aspirin or related medications. Although it is a relatively uncommon disorder, many people with extrinsic asthma and rhinosinusitis will experience some degree of allergic reaction to aspirin when tested.

Deviated Nasal Septum

The nasal septum is a structure made of cartilage that separates the two nostrils of the nose. Although the nasal septum is rarely completely straight, when it becomes significantly bent or buckled, it is known as a "deviated nasal septum." There are several causes for a deviated septum. Some people are born with this condition, or it may develop as a child grows. Other people have a deviated septum due to an injury, generally a broken nose. Although this condition is seldom life threatening, problems may occur because of it. Those with a deviated septum may become more aware of the normal cycle of alternating congestion and decongestion of each side of the nose (nasal cycle), or have persistent blockage of one or both of the nostrils, which can predispose them to infection in the sinuses. Frequent nosebleeds may also occur and noisy breathing or snoring may result. Although a nasal septal deviation may be bothersome, it is not serious. On the other hand, similar symptoms of nasal obstruction and bleeding may be caused by a tumor in the nose. So, when these symptoms increase over time, they should be checked by an otolaryngologist to make sure that they are indeed the result of a septal deviation and not another cause.

Today, a surgical procedure called a septoplasty can be performed, generally on an outpatient basis, to correct this condition. We will discuss this further in Chapter 13.

9

COMPLICATIONS

What Happens if Sinusitis is Not Treated Properly

IN MOST INSTANCES, PEOPLE WITH SINUSITIS either get well without treatment or respond well to antibiotics (assuming it is a bacterial infection). However, in some cases, if they fail to get medical attention or, despite antibiotics, continue to have symptoms, complications can occur. Complications are most likely to occur in children, people with compromised immune systems, such as people with HIV/AIDS or untreated diabetes, or people undergoing chemotherapy.

Although the chances of developing complications are slight if, after two to three weeks your rhinosinusitis is not getting better on its own or does not respond to the treatment, or if it continues to get worse after a few days of treatment prescribed by your doctor, you should seek prompt medical attention. Some of the symptoms to look for include swelling around the eye, double vision, a worsening headache, neck stiffness, nausea, and vomiting. In general, complications are more likely to occur in someone who has not had prior sinusitis, because a person with chronically thickened, inflamed mucus membranes is provided with some degree of protection from complications.

Complications that May Be Related to Sinusitis

LOSS OF SENSE OF SMELL (ANOSMIA). Sinusitis can affect the sense of smell in two ways. Most commonly, it causes swelling of the mucosa lining the nose, thereby reducing the odorants that can reach the olfactory nerve endings high within the nose. This form of anosmia is common, and resolves itself when the sinusitis is treated. However, over time, prolonged nasal and sinus inflammation can also damage the olfactory nerve endings and lead to a permanently reduced sense of smell, or even complete loss. A viral infection or a head injury can occasionally also result in anosmia. Recently, some evidence has been published that certain zinc compounds used to treat viral infections may also result in olfactory loss.

MENINGITIS. Meningitis is an inflammation of the membranes (meninges) and cerebrospinal fluid surrounding the brain and spinal cord. Meningitis may be caused by a virus, fungus, or bacteria and is often a secondary infection—that is, an infection that started somewhere else in the body and traveled through the bloodstream to the brain.

In general, meningitis caused by bacteria is more serious than meningitis caused by a virus. Since a bacterial infection in the sinuses can sometimes lead to meningitis, it is important to understand this disease and to be able to recognize its symptoms.

The most common type of meningococcal meningitis is not caused by sinus disease, but is a contagious illness occurring in children and adolescents, although adults can get it, too. It often spreads quickly in places where many people live together, such as a college dormitory. Because it is most common among children, meningitis can also spread quickly in a school or daycare center. At the outset, this type of meningitis may have many of the same symptoms as influenza, including high fever and headache. What distinguishes its symptoms from those of the flu is that they may also include vomiting, stiff neck, confusion, seizures, tiredness, skin rash, sensitivity to light (photophobia), and small hemorrhages under the skin. In infants, symptoms may include a bulge in the soft spot on the head, unusual irritability, and spasms.

Meningitis caused by sinusitis is not infectious, but occurs because the infection within the sinuses starts to irritate the meninges and then may directly infect them. This type of meningitis usually begins with an acute sinusitis, but instead of getting better, there is a worsening headache, stiff neck, lethargy, and sensitivity to light. Meningitis from a sinus infection is very rare, but can occur at any age. However, the highest incidence is in adolescent males. The reasons for this are not fully understood, although we do know that people without prior sinus infections are at greater risk, and it is possible that estrogen (a female hormone) provides some degree of protection by slightly thickening the sinus mucous membrane.

Although most people recover from meningitis, in 10 to 20 percent of cases it is fatal, so it is always considered a medical emergency. If left untreated, meningitis can also result in a brain abscess or in permanent neurological defects and behavior problems.

Infectious meningitis can be prevented by vaccination, and widespread vaccination for this type of meningitis is now recommended, particularly in college-age adolescents. With meningitis caused by a sinus infection, the initial treatment is usually antibiotics and emergency drainage of the infected sinuses. Medical treatment is then continued until the meningitis has resolved and the sinuses have returned to normal.

ORBITAL CELLULITIS. Orbital cellulitis occurs when infection in one of the sinuses spreads into the eye sockets (orbital periosteum). It is much more common in children than in adolescents and adults. It results in very swollen eyelids (typically just around one eye) and, if it progresses, the swelling alone may temporarily impair vision. Orbital cellulitis must be treated aggressively with antibiotics on an emergency basis, and the eye needs to be carefully observed to ensure that its movement does not become impaired (resulting in double vision), or that the vision in the infected eye does not become more significantly affected, because these can be signs of abscess formation. A CT or MRI scan is often performed to ensure that an early abscess is not present. If the infection does go on to abscess formation, it is usually drained, although in small children (younger than 2 years of age) even abscesses will sometimes resolve with a high dose intravenous antibiotics.

OSTEOMYELITIS. If an infection in the sinus cavities spreads to its bony walls, the result can be osteomyelitis. This is a very rare complication of sinusitis today, but was quite common before antibiotics were discovered. The most common manifestation, marked forehead swelling, was described in 1760 by Sir Percival Pott, a well-known physician in London, and the swelling received the moniker "Potts Puffy Tumor," a name by which it is still known to this day. The swelling is tender, and often red and inflamed, and is treated with antibiotics, surgical drainage, and, occasionally, removal of the inflamed bone.

MUCOCELES. Sinus mucoceles are actually expanded, fluid-filled sinuses. They occur when a sinus is chronically obstructed and fluid continues to build up inside it, causing it to expand. Although frequently referred to as "cysts," mucoceles are very different from the much more common sinus cyst, which is really just a collection of fluid within one area of the lining of the sinus. Sinus cysts rarely cause symptoms or other problems, and are primarily a demonstration that there has either been some sinus inflammation or allergy. Simple sinus cysts are usually not treated unless they are unusual in appearance or grow very large and need to be biopsied.

On the other hand, mucoceles usually grow slowly and expand the sinus and thin its walls and, if left untreated, may cause damage to neighboring structures such as the eye or the brain. Mucocles can result from an injury, a scar, or a tumor, and should be surgically drained. If they become infected, they can grow rapidly all of a sudden, causing other complications, such as headache or orbital pain.

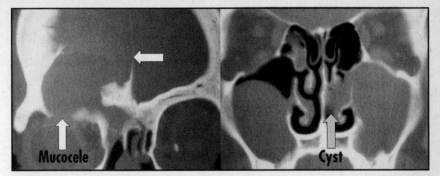

Figure 16. *These CT scans show the presence of a mucocele in the sinus on the left and cysts on the right. Although commonly referred to as "cysts," mucoceles—expanded fluid-filled sinuses—are very different from a sinus cyst, which is really just a collection of fluid within one area of the sinus lining. The mucocele on the left has expanded into the area of the brain (arrows). The cyst in one of the maxillary sinus has also extended into the nose.*

SEPTICEMIA. Septicemia is a very serious, rapidly progressing, life-threatening system-wide infection that occurs when an infection in any part of the body spreads throughout the rest of the body. Untreated, septicemia can cause shock and death. However, it is extremely rare with sinusitis. One type of septicemia is the "toxic shock syndrome" that became well recognized a number of years ago from the use of certain types of tampons. Occasionally, a similar type of toxic shock syndrome can occur from the use of nasal packing following surgery, although it is very rare, since patients are typically treated with antibiotics when packing is in the nose. Symptoms include a very high fever, rapid heart beat, and a rash. People with septicemia are usually placed in the intensive care unit of a hospital and treated with broad spectrum antibiotics. A recently FDA-approved drug, Xigris® (drotrecogin afla), shows great promise in the treatment of septicemia.

ATROPHIC RHINITIS (OZENA). Atrophic rhinitis is another disease that was common before antibiotics were discovered, and is now encountered much more commonly in developing countries than in the United States and Europe. Whereas crusting of the mucus in the front of the nose is relatively common and occurs in many people, particularly during the winter months, in atrophic rhinitis the crusting occurs throughout the nose and is associated with a profuse and sometimes foul-smelling discharge. Although the underlying cause of atrophic rhinitis is not fully understood, it is likely caused by very long-standing and poorly treated sinusitis in which, over time, the underlying bone begins to "melt away," causing more widely open nasal passages. In atrophic rhinitis, the mucous glands in the mucus membrane that lines the nose do not function properly, and thick crusts of dried mucus may build up throughout the nose. This buildup is not only uncomfortable, but may affect a person's sense of smell and cause nosebleeds. Treatment of fully-developed atrophic rhinitis is difficult, and may involve both oral and intravenous antibiotics, as well as surgery to remove any sites of infection. The crusting is significantly helped by the use of nasal irrigations, particularly those containing medicines to soften the crusts.

INVERTED PAPILLOMA. This is the most common form of nasal tumor. It is benign, and usually occurs in adults, typically causing increased nasal obstruction on one side of the nose, occasionally associated with bleeding. The exact cause of this type of tumor is not known, but it is closely associated with the papilloma virus (the same type of virus that causes warts), and there is also an association with chronic sinus inflammation. Although benign, this tumor must be removed because, if it continues to grow, it can affect the eye and the brain and even become life-threatening. Additionally, about 10 to 15 percent of these tumors may harbor a small area of cancer within them. Treatment is surgical removal, and can often be accomplished endoscopically. However, it is important that is the tumor be removed by someone skilled in this type of surgery. If it is not totally removed, the incidence of the tumor recurring (approximately 10 percent) increases dramatically, and the recurrence rate following a second surgery is significantly higher (about 25 percent). Surgery then becomes much more difficult.

ANTIBIOTIC RESISTANCE. Because antibiotics are so effective against bacterial infections, they are now frequently prescribed for a wide variety of illnesses and for patients of all ages. Unfortunately, over the years, some types of bacteria, such as the bacteria that cause tuberculosis, have mutated and are now resistant to the antibiotics that so effectively eliminated them in the past. Even though new types of antibiotics are always being developed, there is still concern among physicians and researchers that overuse of antibiotics or the use of antibiotics for illnesses upon which they have no effect (for example, treating a cold, which is a viral infection), will lead even common bacteria into becoming more rapidly resistant to most or all currently available antibiotics. Since some antibiotic resistance is inevitable, if possible, it is important to limit the use of antibiotics to only those situations in which they are really necessary.

Conditions of the Nose and Face Not Related to Sinusitis

Because the nose and face contain so many organs and systems in such a confined space, it is often difficult for the lay person to understand their interrelationship. In the first part of this chapter, some of the complications that may arise from untreated sinusitis or sinusitis that does not respond to conventional treatment have been discussed. Before leaving this chapter, it is also important to discuss briefly a few conditions that are often thought to be related to sinusitis, but which have very different causes.

NOSEBLEED. Nosebleeds, while often frightening, are usually not serious from a medical standpoint. Nosebleeds may be caused by injury to the nose due to a blow received in a sports competition or an accident. A nosebleed can also be caused by picking at the nose with your fingers. They may also occur during the winter when the air is dry and particularly when the lining of the nose is inflamed following a recent cold. People who take aspirin are also at a higher risk of nosebleeds. Aspirin thins the blood, and that is why it is often prescribed for someone at risk for cardiac disease. If you are taking aspirin and begin to have recurrent nosebleeds, you should discuss with your doctor whether the aspirin should be discontinued. Sometimes people with hypertension (high blood pressure) experience nosebleeds when the pressure within the circulatory system is high enough to rupture the small vessels in the nose.

Because alcohol dilates blood vessels, heavy drinkers may also experience frequent nosebleeds, as may those who are using certain other medications including topical nasal steroids. Those who inhale cocaine may also experience recurrent nosebleeds. The best way to stop a nosebleed is sit down, relax, and either hold the nose, or gently breathe through it, allowing the blood to run down the back of the throat. A topical nasal decongestant (such as Afrin nasal spray) or an icepack held on the back of the neck may also be helpful. The vast majority of nosebleeds, even when they appear profuse, stop with this type of treatment. However, if a nosebleed does not stop within ten minutes or so, it may be wise to have it looked at in the emergency room. Also, if nosebleeds occur frequently, it is wise to consult a doctor. Nasal endoscopy may reveal the site of bleeding, making it possible to cauterize the site. Additionally, nasal endoscopy will allow the unlikely possibility of a more serious condition to be ruled out.

RHINOPHYMA. This condition, characterized by a nose that is abnormally large and bulbous and purplish in color, occurs when the outer layer of skin on the nose thickens. People have long assumed that this condition is limited to people who consume large quantities of alcohol and cartoons that show alcoholics often show the person with this condition. Because alcohol dilates the blood vessels in the nose, extensive alcohol use may, in fact, be a factor in some people, but commonly rhinophyma is much more closely linked to a skin disorder called rosacea. There is no connection between sinusitis and rhinophyma, which is usually treated by surgery, although avoiding heavy alcohol consumption is also usually recommended.

CANCER. Cancer is certainly one of the most dreaded words in the English language, and a diagnosis all of us hope we will never receive. The good news is, however, that today most cancers can be treated, and many people with cancer can be cured.

While all the cells in our body grow by dividing in a manner regulated by our genes, sometimes cells begin to divide abnormally (mutate) and start to invade nearby tissue. Cancer (carcinoma) is the general term for this abnormal and uncontrolled growth of cells.

Although we know with some certainty how cancer works, there are still many theories as to what causes cancer, from the highly scientific to the totally bizarre. We do know that there is a definite link between cancer and the prolonged or intense exposure to radiation and some chemicals (known as carcinogens). And, despite what some tobacco companies claim, the medical community is convinced that there is a link between tobacco use and cancer. Years of research have also shown that certain cancers seem to be caused by viruses although, because there are so many kinds of viruses and so many kinds of cancers, finding the specific virus that causes a specific cancer is an ongoing effort. On the other hand, there is no reason to believe that cancer is caused by high-tension wires, microwave ovens, television signals, or the host of other things you may read about in tabloid newspapers.

In the nose, benign tumors are much more common than malignant (cancerous) tumors. Some factors that may predispose an individual to nasal cancer are known. For instance, it has long been recognized that carpenters working with, and inhaling, hardwood dust are at greater risk of nasal cancer. On the other hand, nasal polyps, unlike polyps in the bowel or stomach, do not predispose a person to the development of cancer. There is also no reason to suspect that cancer in the sinuses is caused by the bacterial or viral infections that generally cause sinusitis.

While cancer was once thought to be a single disease, we now know that there are many different kinds of cancer which affect different parts of the body. Some cancers grow very slowly, others grow and spread very quickly. As a result, some cancers (such as prostate cancer, when diagnosed in very elderly men) are often best left untreated. Other cancers, particularly those that spread quickly (metastisize), are often treated very aggressively with chemotherapy, radiation, surgery, or a combination of all three. There are also many alternative treatments for cancer. Diagnosis and treatment of cancer is individual, and depends on the location and nature of the cancer as well as the age and health of the patient.

The following are examples of different types of cancer that may occur in the head, neck, and sinuses. Most are managed with a combination of surgery and highly focused radiation treatment with, or without, the use of chemotherapy.

SQUAMOUS CELL CANCER. This cancer arises from the skin or squamous mucosa. It is usually treated with a combination of surgery and radiation therapy.

ADENOCARCINOMA. This cancer occurs in the glands of the mucosal lining. In the sinuses, if it is discovered early, surgery combined with radiation therapy is usually very effective.

SARCOMA. Sarcomas are cancers that attack the connective tissues of the body, including fat, muscle, blood vessels, deep skin tissues, nerves, bones, and cartilage. Sarcomas in the sinuses or elsewhere in the head and neck are usually treated with chemotherapy or radiation.

LETHAL MIDLINE GRANULOMA. This rare cancer usually involves the nose and paranasal sinuses. It is really a type of lymphatic cancer and, if left untreated, can cause death by spreading into the central nervous system. Lethal midline granuloma is usually treated with radiation.

MELANOMA. Melanoma is skin cancer, and begins in the skin pigment melanin. It is most commonly experienced by people who have had significant exposure to the sun over many years. However, the reasons why it may occur within the nose and sinuses are less clear. Skin melanoma can be fatal but, if detected early, it is often curable.

10

NONSURGICAL TREATMENT

An Overview of Nonmedical Therapies

S INUSITIS IS OFTEN TREATED WITH MEDICATION, AND IN Chapter 11 we will discuss the relative merits of various prescription and over-the-counter drugs. In Chapter 12, we will discuss some of the so-called alternative medications and therapies now available on the market. In Chapter 13, we will discuss surgical options. Although many medications and surgeries are highly effective in treating infections or complications brought on by sinusitis, often the symptoms can be alleviated by other methods. As we discussed in Chapter 9, continued use of antibiotics may result in antibiotic resistance so, if other remedies can be found, they should also be considered so that use of antibiotics can be limited to only the most severe cases of sinusitis. Recent work suggests that topical nasal steroids may be more effective than antibiotics (in this case amoxicillin) in the treatment of some forms of acute rhinosinusitis.

Solving Other Problems First

TREATING RELATED DISEASES. Because other diseases are often linked to rhinosinusitis, effectively treating these diseases should also help relieve at least some of the symptoms of rhinosinusitis. As you will see in the following section of this chapter, many of the suggested treatments for these related diseases are quite similar to those treatments suggested for rhinosinusitis.

ALLERGIES. As mentioned earlier, people can be allergic to just about anything, and the allergies may be seasonal (usually due to pollen) or perennial (frequently due to dust, molds, or possibly pets). Symptoms include sneezing, runny or stuffy nose, and itchy, watery eyes.

As the years go by, persistent allergies may lead to chronically hyperreactive nasal mucous membranes. In this situation, the patient begins to feel as though he or she is allergic to everything, and things such as temperature change and exposure to perfumes result in nasal congestion and obstruction. It becomes quite bothersome to the patient, but the other classic allergy symptoms tend to disappear.

Most allergies are treated by over-the-counter antihistamines or decongestants, and eyedrops. When these do not work, a topical nasal steroid spray or a prescription antihistamine may be recommended. Allergy testing lets the patient know what environmental factors he or she should avoid. Allergy densensitization (shots) are typically reserved for patients who cannot avoid their allergens, and when other medical therapies do not control the symptoms.

ASTHMA. Asthma is a chronic disorder in which the lungs become inflamed and constricted when exposed to such substances as pollen, dust, mites, and air pollution. The result is wheezing, coughing, and a feeling of tightness in the chest. Classic asthma symptoms include coughing and difficulty breathing. Asthma is treated by prescription drugs, inhalers, and anti-inflammatory corticosteroids or noncorticosteroids, usually under the direction of a pulmonologist or other health care provider.

THE COMMON COLD. Because colds are caused by viruses, there is still very little that can be done to cure a cold. The symptoms of colds such as a stuffy or runny nose, sneezing, coughing, watery eyes, aches and pains, and occasional fever can, however, be alleviated by the use of prescription or over-the-counter decongestants, bed rest, drinking fluids, inhaling steam and/or taking pain killers, such as aspirin, ace-tominophen (Tylenol®), ibuprofen (Advil®, Motrin®), or naproxen (Aleve®). If a cold is persistent or particularly severe, it is a good idea to see a doctor, because a cold may develop into rhinosinusitis.

INFLUENZA AND SARS. Like a cold, influenza is a viral infection, but influenza differs from a cold in that symptoms often include fever, headache, weakness, and fatigue. Influenza is a particularly dangerous disease for the very elderly or people who are already ill or whose immune system is compromised, since influenza can lead to bronchi-tis or pneumonia. Fortunately, vaccines are now available and annual flu vaccination is recommended for most because new strains of influenza develop on a regular basis. Symptoms of influenza may be treated with basically the same medications and therapies as those recommended for the common cold.

The symptoms of SARS can initially be very similar to those of influenza and, although it is under control in most parts of the world now, it is likely to return. Annual flu vaccination therefore could avoid the possibility of being misdiagnosed as a potential case of SARS.

CYSTIC FIBROSIS. Cystic fibrosis is a recessive genetic disorder of the exocrine glands, which produce such bodily secretions as sweat, mucus, and enzymes, and which affects the lungs, digestive, and reproductive systems. Those who have cystic fibrosis experience a continuous buildup of mucus in the lungs that often results in frequent infections and often lung damage. There is no cure for cystic fibrosis and, in the past, those with it rarely survived beyond childhood. Now, however, with early diagnosis, many people with cystic fibrosis are living into middle age through a combination of physiotherapy, enzyme replacement, antibiotic therapy, vitamins, careful attention to diet, and inhalation therapy.

GASTROESOPHAGEAL REFLUX DISEASE. The esophagus is, strictly speaking, a part of the gastrointestinal system and not part of the respiratory system. However, because mucus produced in the nose passes down the esophagus into the stomach, the esophagus is clearly affected if there is any disease in the sinuses. Likewise, the sinuses can be impacted by any problems that occur in the esophagus.

The most common of these is gastroesophageal reflux disease (GERD), or heartburn. When a person is suffering from GERD, the acid produced in the stomach refluxes (backs up) into the esophagus, often to the extent that it reaches the mouth. While almost everyone experiences episodes of heartburn occasionally, the lining of the esophagus usually offers enough protection from the acid so that little harm is done. If, one the other hand, reflux occurs on a regular basis, the lining of the esophagus can become severely damaged.

There is some evidence that GERD in children may be a cause of sinusitis. Children tend to experience GERD more often than adults, and are more likely to have colds that result in coughing, throat irritation, and infection. If adults experience GERD on a regular basis, the acid refluxed may irritate the lining of the pharynx, leading to infection. Chronic GERD should be treated to avoid problems with either the esophagus or inflammation in the larynx (laryngitis and cough).

In most cases, treatment for GERD involves elevating the head of the bed six inches or so, not eating food within two hours of going to bed, and avoiding certain foods like tomato products, acidic beverages like orange juice, and caffeine. It is also generally recommended that those suffering from GERD avoid alcohol, carbonated beverages, and unusually spicy foods. If symptoms persist, one of many over-the-counter antacids may be effective. If those don't work, there are also many effective prescription medications including proton pump inhibitors (which decrease the production of stomach acid) and histamine acid (H2) blockers. Surgery is another option. An evaluation by a gastroenterologist is recommended to rule out a more serious condition and to evaluate the necessity of surgical option.

Treating Rhinosinusitis

HYDRATION. The good news for many rhinosinusitis sufferers is that one of the most widely used and economical treatments is one of Earth's most freely available substances—water. In treatment of rhinosinusitis, water may be used in several ways.

DRINKING PLENTY OF WATER. There is now some question as to whether all people actually need to drink the eight glasses of water that have been recommended for years as part of a healthy lifestyle (and a key to many weight-loss programs). However, it is probably still true that those suffering from a cold or rhinosinusitis should drink plenty of it. Why does drinking water help?

The human body is between 50 and 60 percent water, depending on the age and sex of the individual. Babies are about 75 percent water, while older people may be in the range of 45 percent water and, in general, young men are composed of about 10 percent more water than young women. The rest of us are somewhere in between. While the lungs contain the most water of any of the organs of the body (about 80 percent of the lung tissue is water), water is also an important component of all cells. Each individual cell, like the lungs, are about 80 percent water. Water is also an integral component of mucus. The body excretes about a liter of water a day through the skin, lungs, kidneys, and through excreting feces and urine, blowing one's nose, or sweating.

Because water is essential to life, not surprisingly, one of the major functions of the body is to achieve a fluid balance—that is, to make sure that the amount of water excreted does not exceed the amount of water taken in. In a normal, healthy human, consuming water when thirsty usually achieves this balance. When a person has a cold or acute or chronic rhinosinusitis, however, a more than an average amount of fluid is lost. And, when the body does not get enough water, mucus tends to thicken. Therefore, an above average amount of water must be taken in to maintain fluid balance and to help lubricate the mucous membranes, thereby helping the cilia to clear the mucus.

Although any fluid contains at least some water, some fluids, such as alcoholic beverages and coffee, actually dehydrate the system. Water of any temperature will have the same effect in rehydrating the body but a hot beverage such as tea or soup has the additional advantage of providing steam that may also help relieve congestion. While any soup will provide this effect, there is actually some scientific evidence to suggest that chicken soup, just like your mother may have told you, may be the best way to treat rhinosinusitis. Since chicken is a protein, it contains animo acids, which are chemically similar to acetylcystine, an ingredient in drugs commonly prescribed for respiratory infections. Chicken soup inhibits the migration of inflammatory white blood cells and lessens the inflammatory effect of rhinoviruses.

INHALING STEAM. In addition to consuming water, many rhinosinusitis sufferers find significant relief from symptoms by inhaling steam, which acts as an expectorant, that is, something that softens mucus, and makes you cough or spit.

The easiest and most economical way to inhale steam is to fill a bowl with hot water and simply lean over the bowl and inhale. Some people find that they are able to inhale more steam if they put a towel over their head and the bowl so that the steam does not escape as quickly into the surrounding air. Generally, a person should inhale steam in this manner for 10 minutes or so to achieve the best effect.

(Note: Avoid inhaling steam from a kettle or pan in which water is still boiling as the steam is hot enough to burn your skin and injure the delicate lining of your nose.) While steam alone can greatly relieve rhinosinusitis symptoms, additional beneficial effects may be obtained by adding menthol or eucalyptus oil to the water. Menthol and eucalyptus can provide some anti-inflammatory relief, as well as acting as expectorants.

The same effect may be achieved from taking a long, hot shower. A hot shower has the additional advantage of helping to massage and soothe the aching muscles many people experience if they have a cold.

VAPORIZERS AND HUMIDIFIERS. Vaporizers and humidifiers offer another option for inhaling steam. Both are machines that produce water vapor. Humidifiers produce mist; vaporizers produce warm mist.

Although vaporizers and humidifiers are clearly helpful in some disorders (for instance, croup in children) and they may helpful in relieving the symptoms of an acute upper respiratory tract infection, their role in the treatment of chronic rhinosinusitis is less clear. To be effective in raising the humidity of a room, they need to be left running over a prolonged period of time and this, unfortunately, may increase the risk of molds in the atmosphere.

Warm mist vaporizers have the advantage of putting more water vapor into the air. A cool mist humidifier is not able to produce as much water vapor as a warm mist vaporizer, but may be safer. Many of the newer models contain filters that help eliminate the growth of fungi and bacteria but, even if it has a filter, a vaporizer or humidifier must be cleaned often, so it is less likely to provide an environment in which molds, fungi, and bacteria can live.

Depending on brand name and various features, most vaporizers or humidifiers cost from between $25 and $150, and can be purchased at most pharmacies, hardware stores, department stores, or on the Internet. A listing of the various humidifiers available, their features and prices may be found on the Internet at AllergyBuyersClub.com.

In general, when shopping for a vaporizer or humidifier, look for a unit that is easy to handle (some are quite heavy when full of water) and easy to clean, with removable parts that can be washed in a dishwasher. It should also be safe, particularly if it is to be used in a household where small children are present.

Those who live in a climate that is cold in the winter and hot in the summer generally find that heating and air conditioning are important factors in relieving the symptoms of rhinosinusitis. However, air conditioning and heating ducts can become contaminated with mold, and this can be a source of irritation for people with mold allergies. Additionally, heating and air conditioning systems, while making the interior of a home or office a comfortable temperature, unfortunately also dry the air that we breathe considerably. Humidifiers and vaporizers can alleviate symptoms by providing moisture but, as stated above, if not cleaned conscientiously, can also harbor fungi, bacteria, and molds.

USE OF GENTLE, MOIST HEAT. When the sinus cavities are swollen and inflamed, many rhinosinusitis sufferers find that the application of a warm moist cloth to the face offers some relief to the symptoms they are experiencing. While such a remedy will not cure the sinusitis, the warmth of the cloth may make the sufferer feel better and the moisture that is inhaled may help to moisten the mucous membranes in the nose.

MEDICATED RUBS. The use of medicated vapor rubs to alleviate cold symptoms goes back thousands of years, but is still an effective remedy for many rhinosinusitis sufferers. Most vapor rubs contain either menthol or eucalyptus and are available in creams or oils designed to be rubbed onto the chest so that the vapors are easily inhaled. Medicated rubs are generally used at bedtime to help you breathe easily while sleeping. In addition, since they produce a fairly strong odor, you would probably not want to use them while in school or at a work environment.

Medicated rubs are available at pharmacies, natural food stores, and on the Internet and cost about $5 for 3 ounces. If you use medicated rubs, it is important to remember, however, that they should not be rubbed inside the nose or mouth, since they may irritate the mucous membranes.

SALINE SPRAYS. Saline sprays, sometimes also known as ocean sprays (because they contain salt water), also provide symptom relief to sufferers of rhinosinusitis. Saline sprays, if used properly, can both reduce thickened mucus in the nose and assist in the removal of infectious agents such as mold, fungi and bacteria. In most patients, saline sprays can be used up to six times a day, although it is always a good idea to consult your doctor before you try any remedy, as each person's situation is different.

Saline sprays can be either isotonic or hypertonic. Isotonic solutions have a similar amount of salt to that present in the cells of the body. Hypertonic saline, on the other hand, has more salt than is present in body cells. Hypertonic saline tends to burn and, in the short term, may make the cilia beat faster and increase their ability to clear mucus. However, there is also a real concern that in the long run these may damage the mucus membranes and perhaps should be avoided.

There are many saline sprays on the market and, depending on whether they come premixed in a container that can be used to apply the spray, they cost from about $5 to $30. However, it is also easy to make saline spray yourself. The most effective recipe for saline spray is one cup of cooled boiled water, 1/4 teaspoon of non-iodized salt, and 1/4 teaspoon of baking soda. It is important to boil the water you use in a saline spray to remove impurities and as much contamination as possible. The addition of the baking soda (which is a base, or alkaline, substance) helps counteract the acidity in the spray.

It is also important that the homemade saline solution is fresh and not stored more than 4 to 7 days even in a refrigerator, as it will become contaminated with bacteria. Similarly, the device used to dispense the salt water must be either boiled or washed in very hot water before the saline is poured into it. Saline sprays that are pre-mixed and prepackaged sometimes contain the preservative benzalkonium chloride (BKC). In general, it is probably best to avoid solutions containing BKC, since some studies have shown that BKC can damage the mucous membranes, decrease movement of mucus by the cilia, and inhibit neutrophil function. (Neutrophils are produced by the immune system and attack foreign substances such as bacteria.)

To use a prepackaged saline nasal spray you should first blow your nose to clear it. Then, tilt your head slightly forward, close the side of the nose not receiving the spray, squeeze the bottle gently and begin to breathe in slowly through your nose. A homemade saline spray can be applied using a plastic bottle with a nozzle attached that produces a mist. To apply the spray, simply place the nozzle at the entrance of the nostril and gently squeeze the bottle and inhale. Do not place the nozzle up into the nose.

Because saline sprays do not contain medications, and because they are similar to the composition of the water in your body, there is no risk of becoming addicted to them.

SALINE IRRIGATION. Saline irrigation works on the same principle as saline spray. The only difference is that, rather than a mist, irrigation involves a gentle stream of saline solution. There are many nasal irrigation products on the market and they range from about $20 to $150. The more expensive machines feature a small compressor unit with a handheld wand. Units such as the Waterpik® may include a nasal adapter. Soft nasal adapters are also available, which may be slipped into the nasal cavity and produce a fine spray. You can also use a dental syringe with a small bulb on the end and apply the saline solution by compressing the bulb. A small catheter or nasal douche is also effective. Typically about 1/4 to 1/2 cup is recommended for each nostril. Another unit, the SinuNEB®, provides nebulized saline or medications accessory for daily nasal cleaning with saline.

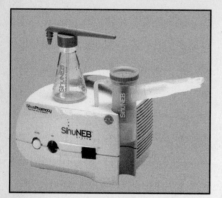

Figure 17. *The SinuNEB system is a prescription intranasal nebulized therapy. An irrigator attachment, shown sitting on top of the SinuNEB compressor, is supplied for daily nasal irrigation/cleaning with saline solution in addition to the nebulizer attachment, shown on the right, that patients use for medication application.*

No matter what type of irrigation method you use, you must be very diligent about cleaning the device to make sure that bacteria, fungi, and mold do not grow in it. If you hand wash your irrigator, you should use diluted bleach. You can also boil the components of the irrigation system or wash them in the dishwasher. Of course, you should always follow the manufacturer's recommended cleaning steps whenever possible to insure the product is not damaged during cleaning.

EATING SPICY FOODS. Virtually everyone, rhinosinusitis sufferer or not, has experienced how hot, spicy foods can cause the eyes to water and the nose to run. While hot, spicy foods may temporarily clear the sinuses, they may compound the problem in people who suffer from GERD or food allergies.

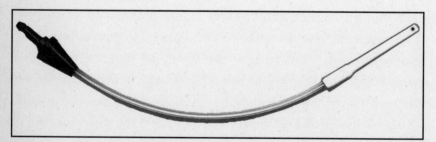

Figure 18. *Ethicare's DSI, a flexible sinus flush irrigator, is designed to provide a steady liquid solution flow that reaches hard-to-irrigate places, particularly after surgery. It directly irrigates in the hard-to-reach crevices in the nasal passage, as well as into the sinus if an opening is left by sinus surgery.*

11

THE ROLE OF ANTI-INFECTIVE MEDICATIONS IN TREATING SINUSITIS

When Home Remedies Are Not Enough

As SOON AS OTHER CAUSES FOR THE SYMPTOMS have been ruled out, and a diagnosis of sinusitis has been made, it is time to consider what, if any, medications would be appropriate. In some cases, treatments such as inhaling steam, applying a vapor rub, using saline sprays or irrigation, installing a vaporizer or humidifier, or simply drinking more water might alleviate symptoms. However, if the symptoms persist, an over-the-counter or prescription medication, or combination of medications, may be indicated.

Because acute, recurrent, and chronic rhinosinusitis may have a variety of causes, the first step in determining what treatment would be most effective is to isolate the cause of the distress. As we discussed in Chapter 1, rhinosinusitis is an inflammation of the mucous membranes lining any of the nasal and sinus cavities. Inflammation may be caused by a variety of irritants, including air pollution, smoking, climate, allergies, colds, and infections, which may be caused by viruses, bacteria, and fungi. Before you can effectively be treated for your rhinosinusitis, it is important that you and your doctor work together to diagnose and determine what the cause of your rhinosinusitis is, so that the appropriate treatment or medication can be prescribed (Chapter 8).

Treating Acute, Recurrent, or Chronic Rhinosinusitis

The next step in deciding what medication or treatment to prescribe is to determine if the sinusitis is acute, recurrent, or chronic, since medications and treatments may differ, depending on the severity and anticipated duration of the distress.

Acute rhinosinusitis is in many ways the easiest type of the disease to treat with medication. Its symptoms may come on fairly quickly with little warning (such as a previous cold), and may become quite distressing and painful almost immediately. If the patient has never had a sinus infection, the symptoms may easily be confused with a toothache, headache, earache, or pain in the eyes or cheeks. Since acute rhinosinusitis is such a common illness, however, most family physicians are able to diagnose it accurately. Treatment may consist of the therapies described in the previous chapter, with the addition of one of the broad-spectrum antibiotics listed later on in this chapter. Those suffering from acute rhinosinusitis generally recover completely within two weeks or so, and may not have another problem with it for months or even years.

Recurrent rhinosinusitis begins with an episode of the acute form of the disease but, instead of being followed by complete recovery and a period free of symptoms, the infection recurs at least several times a year. Because the symptoms are familiar to sufferers, they usually seek medical attention quickly and, within two weeks, generally find relief from antibiotics. One of the problems faced by those with recurrent rhinosinusitis, however, is that, by taking antibiotics on a frequent basis, they may find that the bacteria causing their discomfort become resistant to antibiotics and, sooner or later, they may require either a different kind of antibiotic or other medication. Because antibiotic resistance is a serious problem, it is recommended that those with recurrent rhinosinusitis seek the advice of an otolaryngologist, a specialist in diseases of the sinuses. The sinus specialist can obtain a culture under endoscopic visualization and prescribe an antibiotic, based upon the type of bacteria cultured and its sensitivity to antibiotics. Alternative types of medical treatments or, occasionally, surgery may be recommended.

Chronic rhinosinusitis, by contrast, is a disease that seems to persist for weeks or months at a time, often despite various attempts to treat it with medications or other therapies. Chronic sinusitis may also be the result of damage to the mucus membranes, either from untreated acute sinusitis or repeated bouts of sinusitis that may or may not be caused by the same bacteria, fungi, or viruses. Chronic sinusitis is also associated with other chronic diseases such as cystic fibrosis and asthma. Because chronic rhinosinusitis is a complicated and often stubborn disease, it is generally recommended that those suffering from it see an otolaryngologist. If the strongest medical therapy fails, surgery may be recommended.

Treating Patients with Rhinosinusitis plus Allergies and/or Asthma

Because many sinusitis patients also have allergies, asthma, and some may have Samter's Triad, choosing the appropriate medical therapy is often a complicated process. Obviously, it is important that in treating one disease, the treatment not make other diseases worse. If you suffer from more than one respiratory ailment, it is certainly important that you make your physician aware of your situation. Again, it is probably also a good idea to consult an otolaryngologist and, if allergies or immunologic problems are a factor, specialists may either recommend consultation with an allergist or perform allergy testing themselves.

Although each person's situation may be a bit different, in general, patients with multiple respiratory illnesses are generally treated with environmental control and a combination of antibiotics, anti-inflammatory agents such as corticosteroids, antihistamines, and/or allergy shots. If fungi are playing a part in the inflammation, antifungal medications may also be helpful.

Allergy desensitization (shots) is usually reserved for situations in which it is not possible for someone to avoid the offending allergens, and medical therapy is not providing adequate relief. Allergy shots are dilute solutions of the allergens and, by giving them on a regular basis, the body develops tolerance to these allergens. It is now known that the body actually develops blocking antigens (IgE) during therapy with allergy shots. Usually, allergy shots are initially given once a week and then less frequently when a maintenance level of treatment is reached. Most physicians who treat allergies increase the concentration of the allergens in the shots as tolerance to the shots develops. A typical course of allergy desensitization is approximately two years.

Antibiotics

By the late 1800s, doctors and research scientists began to make the connection between disease and germs, and started searching for medications that would kill bacteria and other disease-causing microbes. Although several European researchers had investigated the germ-disease connection, British scientist Alexander Fleming is generally credited with discovering the first antibiotic, penicillin, in the 1920s. Although penicillin was tested on a number of patients with bacterial infections, it wasn't widely used until World War II, when it was used to treat wounded soldiers. After World War II, it became widely available for treating civilians and, until the late 1950s, was available to the public without a prescription.

Unfortunately, too many people seized upon this new wonder drug as the magic cure-all for just about every ailment, and many strains of bacteria soon became penicillin-resistant. To deal with this problem, scientists formulated other forms of penicillin, including ampicillin. Other types of antibiotics were also discovered, and physicians today have a wide variety of different products to consider when prescribing an antibiotic.

HOW DO ANTIBIOTICS WORK? As we have discussed earlier in the book, the body is literally packed with different types of bacteria. In fact, without bacteria, such as the bacteria (for example, the kind that help us digest our food), we could not survive. However, not all bacteria are beneficial to us. When disease-causing bacteria get into our bodies they begin to invade our healthy cells, causing us to get infections. Penicillin works by preventing cell wall synthesis. The bacteria cannot form normal cell walls, and they die. Other types of antibiotics kill bacteria by interrupting or slowing down the bacteria's reproduction and functioning.

WHY ARE THERE SO MANY KINDS OF ANTIBIOTICS? In addition to type of penicillin, doctors may now choose among cephalosporins, tetracyclines, aminoglycosides, quinolones, macrolides, and others. The advantage of having so many types of antibiotics available is that physicians now have the opportunity to choose the antibiotic that specifically targets the bacteria that are causing the disease. Penicillins, cephalosporins, and related compounds are in a classification of antibiotics known as beta-lactams, because they work by interfering with the cell walls of bacteria. Beta-lactams are particularly effective against the kinds of bacteria that cause pneumonia and that infect the upper respiratory tract.

Macrolides and azalides are also often used in patients with upper respiratory infections and are particularly useful for patients who are allergic to penicillins.

Trimethoprim-sulfamethoxazole may still be used for patients with acute sinusitis and, in chronic sinusitis, may be used in conjunction with another antibiotic to provide broad spectrum bacterial coverage. It has the advantage of being less expensive than amoxicillin and also provides an alternative for those who are allergic to penicillin.

Quinolones act by interfering with the bacteria's ability to reproduce and are often used to treat adults with chronic sinusitis. One of the quinolones, Cipro®, recently gained widespread publicity when it was prescribed as a treatment for anthrax. In general, the quinolones have a low incidence of intestinal side effects but may cause some other symptoms that are not typically associated with taking antibiotics. These include dizziness, or an increased tendency for tendons and ligaments to pull or tear with heavy exercise.

Lincosamides also prohibit bacteria from reproducing.

Tetracyclines are effective in prohibiting bacterial growth but, unfortunately, have side effects such as skin reaction to sunlight and tooth discoloration.

Ketolides are a new class of antibiotics that have been available in many countries for some time and now are available in the United States, broadening the opportunities to treat sinusitis caused by bacteria that are resistant to other older antibiotics.

ANTIBIOTIC RESISTANCE. Even though there are now dozens of types of antibiotics on the market, unfortunately, there are still not enough. The reason is the phenomenon of antibiotic resistance. Why do bacteria become resistant to antibiotics? Like all living things, bacteria have the ability to mutate, that is, change their genetic structure over time in order to survive. As in other species, in bacteria the strongest survive, creating increasingly more resistant superbugs.

While it can take humans and other more genetically complicated animals thousands of years to evolve, bacteria are relatively short-lived, and the adaptations they make to a hostile environment can occur in months or, at the most, a few years. So, as soon as a new antibiotic is developed, it is likely that sooner or later the bacteria it was designed to kill will begin trying to develop defenses against it.

However unintentionally, we humans often help this process along. Because we live in towns and cities and travel frequently from country to country, we spread not only diseases to one another, but also the types of bacteria that have become resistant to antibiotics. A case in point is the bacteria that cause tuberculosis. In the recent past, tuberculosis was nearly eliminated in the United States. Now, because the bacteria that cause tuberculosis have become so resistant to antibiotics, the disease is less contained than it was decades ago.

Unfortunately, hospitals, the very institutions that are designed to treat disease, have also become centers for the transmission of drug-resistant bacteria. In fact, each year up to two million Americans find that a side effect of their hospital stay was an unwelcome infection of some kind.

Overuse of antibiotics has also contributed to the problem. When antibiotics were first introduced, they were so effective against some diseases that they were prescribed for a host of others, some of which they had no effect upon at all (for example, viral diseases). Yet, patients continued to demand them, and too many doctors continued to prescribe them. This situation may become more serious in the future as more people are beginning to purchase drugs by mail and over the Internet from foreign countries where antibiotics often do not require a prescription.

Noncompliance with prescription dosages is also a contributory factor to antibiotic resistance. Today's antibiotics often work so quickly to alleviate symptoms that, as soon as patients begin to feel better, they stop taking the prescribed dosage. Even though they feel better, they may still have the bacteria present, and these remaining disease-causing bacteria may continue to slowly reproduce, often gaining resistance to the antibiotic in the process.

Some would argue that another significant problem with resistance has been caused by agriculture. On large corporate forms, livestock such as cattle and chickens are raised in close proximity to one another, and diseases can spread quickly in a herd or flock. It is estimated that half of all antibiotics now produced are given to farm animals to prevent disease. Because these antibiotics are given to the animals to protect against infection, they are usually given in low doses, and some bacteria may survive and mutate into resistant forms. Some of the inevitable antibiotic resistance developed in these animals is passed on to the humans who eat them. Legislation is now pending to curb some of this type of antibiotic use.

Unfortunately, despite the introduction of all the various families of antibiotics, there is some form of bacterial resistance to every one of them, making our ability to cure certain infections already very difficult today, with the future being very uncertain and reliant on our ability to continue to find newer and more powerful antibiotics.

WHAT IS A "BROAD SPECTRUM ANTIBIOTIC"? As the name suggests, broad spectrum antibiotics are those antibiotics that have been proven to be effective in attacking a wide range of bacteria. Broad spectrum antibiotics are often prescribed to treat acute rhinosinusitis, since it is often not important to determine specifically what bacteria are causing the infection if the patient is only going to be use the drug rarely. If you are subject to recurrent or chronic rhinosinusitis, however, your doctor may recommend a nasal culture to try to identify the specific bacteria present so that, when an antibiotic is prescribed, it is assured to be active against the bacteria and has not become resistant.

All of us have "good" bacteria in the bowels, which are important in the digestion of food. Broad spectrum antibiotics may kill these "good" bacteria as well as the infection that the antibiotics are treating, allowing other, more resistant, bacteria to take their place in the bowels. These new bacteria, which then colonize the bowels, can cause diarrhea and damage the lining of the bowel. Because of this problem, if you are placed on a broad spectrum antibiotic, it is advisable to also take acidophilus or lactobacillus on a daily basis throughout the duration of the antibiotic therapy and for a few days after it has been finished. This is particularly important when treating chronic rhinosinusitis, because the antibiotic courses often need to be prolonged. Taking acidophilus or lactobacillus helps the bowels maintain the normal flora (that is, the "good" bacteria) when taking antibiotics. Acidophilus and lactobacillus are the bacteria found in live culture yogurt; they are also available in pill form from a pharmacy or health food store.

In any case, if you develop more than a mild diarrhea while taking a broad spectrum antibiotic, it is important to call you doctor. You should not take antidiarrheal medications because, if the diarrhea is due to a change in the bowel flora (that is, disease-causing bacteria), that new bacteria can damage the lining of the bowels. Another type of antibiotic may be necessary to restore the normal bowel flora if the symptoms are not alleviated when the antibiotic that caused the problem is discontinued.

WHICH ANTIBIOTIC IS RIGHT FOR YOU? Before a doctor can determine which antibiotic is right for you, the first question will be whether an antibiotic of any kind can effectively treat your rhinosinusitis. Remember, antibiotics are only effective against infections caused by bacteria. They won't help you if your sinusitis is caused by viruses or fungi or any of the other irritants we've discussed in this chapter. As we've discussed earlier, receiving unnecessary antibiotics can prove harmful to you if overuse or misuse results in resistance. The second question will be whether or not you have allergies to any antibiotics.

Medications for Virus Infections

As you may remember from high school science, bacteria are large enough that you can easily see them in a microscope. Viruses, however, are so tiny that they can only be seen by a specialized instrument called an electron microscope. Unlike bacteria, which are creatures that exist independently, viruses are basically nucleic acid

(RNA or DNA) coated with proteins. They can only multiply inside a living cell.

In addition to the common cold, we know that viruses are responsible for diseases such as polio, influenza, chickenpox, smallpox, herpes cold sores, AIDS, SARS, and Ebola. Most diseases caused by viruses can be transmitted from human to human. In the case of the common cold, hand contact is the most common form of transmission. Of course, cold viruses can be passed on by sneezing or coughing; however, viruses are more frequently transmitted by touching a person or an object where the virus is present. Viruses can also be contracted on surfaces and then, at a later time, transferred to the mucus membranes of the mouth or to the eye by touching or rubbing these areas. Washing your hands is very important in preventing the transmission of the common cold. Some viruses, such as West Nile virus and rabies, can be transmitted to humans from animals. It is suspected that other diseases, such as some kinds of cancer and multiple sclerosis, may also be caused by viruses.

Unfortunately, although we understand how viruses cause disease, as yet we have few medications that can kill viruses and thus cure the diseases they cause, including the colds that often lead to rhinosinusitis.

There are now several very effective vaccines that prevent viral diseases such as polio, chickenpox, smallpox, and influenza. These vaccines consist of killed viruses, and work by prompting the immune system to respond to live viruses of the same type that may enter the body. As yet, however, there are no approved vaccines for the most serious viral infections, such as AIDS, or those that are the most common, such as colds.

Vaccines may also be helpful in combating some bacterial infections. In the year 2000, the U.S. Food and Drug Administration approved the vaccine Prevnar, which can be used to prevent pneumonoccal infections, the leading cause of meningitis, pneumonia, and sometimes the cause of sinus infections, particularly in young children. At present, Prevnar is recommended for children under 2 years of age.

From both the doctor's and patient's points of view, it can sometimes be difficult to differentiate bacterial from viral rhinosinusitis. The nasal discharge may become discolored after a while in a viral infection, without a true bacterial rhinosinusitis being present. X-rays and CT scans are not at all helpful, since they show similar pictures in both. The doctor will typically use a combination of the symptoms, the duration of the infection (viral infections usually start to improve after five to seven days), and a physical examination to try to make this differentiation. Bacterial cultures are definitive, but results take about 48 hours and are, therefore, not practical in a clinical setting when a rapid response is required.

The "electronic nose" is an exciting new technology, which has shown promise in distinguishing bacteria from viruses in the research setting. This electronic device is used in the food industry to sense food that is going bad, as well as being used in some other commercial and bio-defense environments. Research at the University of Pennsylvania has demonstrated that the electronic nose may also help with some common dilemmas in the clinical setting (for example, bacterial versus viral, whether or not to prescribe antibiotics, and so on) by analyzing the patient's breath while diagnosing sinusitis and pneumonia. Given that many viral infections are currently treated with antibiotics because the physician is not sure whether a bacterial infection is present, the potential for a device that can rapidly and easily differentiate bacteria from viruses is of major importance. However, it will require further research and development before this device becomes readily available device for routine testing in the doctor's office.

Fungi

There is considerable controversy surrounding the connection between rhinosinusitis and fungi. Some of the controversy revolves around the issuance of a patent to Drs. Jens Ponikau and the Mayo Clinic in April 2003. The patent issued is a "methods patent," covering the use of antifungal agents to any mucosal surface. This includes topical antifungal agents used in the treatment of chronic rhinosinusitis, otitis media, asthma, and gastroenterological disorders. Surprisingly, this patent was issued despite the fact that topical anti-fungal agents have been in use in several of these areas for many years. Theoretically, the patent blocks anyone (other than the Mayo Clinic) from selling an antifungal agent to treat these conditions without the approval of the Mayo Clinic. Interestingly, no drugs at all—of any type, including antibiotics—have yet been approved by the US Food and Drug Administration (FDA) for the treatment of chronic rhinos-inusitis although, as will be discussed later, many drugs are commonly prescribed for this condition. Even more controversy has been cre-ated by some unwarranted claims, not well backed by scientific stud-ies, regarding the role of fungus and antifungal treatments. Such issues have primarily been presented in the lay press, and include a state-ment by leaders in the Mayo research group that their theories about the role of fungi in the disease process represent "a quantum shift in thinking, similar in magnitude to the discovery by Copernicus that the earth moves around the sun."

More recently, the Mayo Clinic circulated an even more controver-sial patient flyer that claimed that traditional therapies for chronic rhi-nosinusitis, including antibiotics, topical nasal steroids, and endoscopic sinus surgery, are ineffective. This is clearly erroneous and misleading to patients, and contrary to a large body of scientific evidence.

According to Dr. Ponikau, all chronic sinusitis is caused by an immune response to common fungi in the air. Further, Dr. Ponikau and his colleagues, Dr. David Sherris and Dr. Eugene Kern, have stated that their studies indicate that "fungus allergy was thought to be involved in less than ten percent of cases. Our studies indicate that, in fact, fungus is likely the cause of nearly all of these problems. And it is not an allergic reaction, but an immune reaction."

Although the Mayo claims are exaggerated and are based on lim-ited scientific evidence, their work has demonstrated that fungi appear to play a larger a role in this disease process than was previously recognized. Ponikau and others have demonstrated that, if you use careful techniques, you can find fungi in everyone's nose, whether they have rhinosinusitis or not.

However, it appears that in certain individuals with a propensity toward chronic sinusitis, the body may react to fungi in the mucus by sending eosinophils to attack the fungi. It is these eosinophils, the same cells that are frequently seen in an allergic reaction, that irritate the membranes of the nose, increase nasal reactivity, and significantly worsen the chronic rhinosinusitis. Therefore, although there is no scientific basis for the claim that fungi are the cause of all chronic rhinosinusitis, certain patients may indeed benefit from environmental control of fungal exposure, or the use of a topical or an oral antifungal agent. At the time of this writing, properly controlled scientific studies are underway to evaluate the use of antifungal agents in chronic rhinosinusitis. Clarifying the potential role of fungus will be a solid contribution to our understanding of the many factors involved in this disease.

The controversy surrounding the issuance of this very broad methods patent to Mayo, based upon limited scientific evidence, has also raised interest in the lay press. Following a front-page article in *The Wall Street Journal* expressing some surprise about the patent, Donald C. Lanza, M.D., president of the American Rhinologic Society, wrote a follow-up letter that was published in the paper on May 14, 2003 which, in part, read, "Antifungal agents are not new, nor is the concept of topically administering them to the nose. Physicians have been developing new methods for treating patients for generations without obtaining patents. The role of the physician is to pass those methods on to as many other physicians as possible, so that more patients may be effectively treated. While physicians may reasonably differ on the effectiveness of this proposed treatment, it must be recognized that awarding such a patent will potentially create a stranglehold on current and future treatments."

Given that physicians have indeed been using topical antifungal agents in the nose and the upper aero-digestive tract for many years, it appears unlikely that, if challenged, this broad patent will hold. However, it is also true that history will likely not consider this a high point either in either American medicine or in the wisdom of the US Patent Office.

ANTIFUNGAL MEDICATIONS. Both topical and oral antifungal agents have been used to treat chronic rhinosinusitis when a fungus is, or appears to be, a factor in the disease process; however, none have yet been approved by the FDA. The most common oral antifungal medications are Sporanox® (itraconazole) and Lamisil® (terbenifine), although a more recent antifungal (voriconazole) has also been used in some situations. Both Sporanox® and Lamisil® have been approved for the treatment of such fungal conditions as toenail infections, but have not, to date, been proven effective or been approved for the treatment of fungal sinusitis. Indeed, the FDA recently issued a warning about the occasional severe side effects of these medications, as a few cases of liver failure and heart failure have been reported in conjunction with the use of both medications.

However, there is some evidence to suggest that anti-fungal agents are indeed helpful in some difficult-to-treat sinus infections in which fungus plays a role. Unfortunately, in addition to some occasional severe side effects, both these medications are very expensive, and often have to be taken for several months. Insurance companies frequently balk at paying for antifungal agents, ostensibly because they are not approved for this purpose. However, in reality, no antibiotics are approved for use in chronic sinusitis, either, so the difference would appear to be one of cost, not one of FDA approval. Because these medications are so expensive, if they are prescribed and not covered by insurance, some patients have purchased them in Canada or overseas.

Since both antifungal agents have the potential to cause liver toxicity, liver function tests are usually performed before and during treatment, and the medications are not appropriate for people who have liver problems or are on certain other medications. They should also be avoided in a patient with a history of heavy alcohol use or someone with a history of heart failure.

Antifungal agents have also been used topically in nasal irrigation or spray. Unfortunately, some of the medications either do not dissolve or are not very stable in solution. For example, amphotericin B has to be dissolved in water instead of saline, needs to be protected from light, and is only stable for a few days to a week in solution. Nystatin has also been used in nasal irrigation. These medications, used topically, appear to be safe, but their efficacy has not yet been proven.

Generally, oral antifungal therapy is reserved for situations in which there is ample evidence that fungi may be a significant factor in the patient's disease, and if other more conventional therapies have not been effective.

Over-the-Counter Medications

Over-the-counter medications are remedies that do not require a prescription. They may be purchased by anyone at pharmacies, by mail, or on the Internet. Many over-the-counter medications can be quite effective in treating the symptoms of acute rhinosinusitis but, at this point, it is important to raise some cautions. Many over-the-counter medications are combination products, that is, they contain not just one medication, such as an expectorant, but may also contain other ingredients as well, such as a pain reliever. Because those who suffer from rhinosinusitis may be sensitive to some of the ingredients in an over-the-counter medication, it is important that anyone who takes them carefully read the ingredients on the package. Better yet, before taking an over-the-counter medication, it is a good idea to ask your doctor what medications would be most appropriate for your particular illness.

GENERIC DRUGS. Patients are often confused about what generic drugs are, so at this point it is probably appropriate to clear up some misconceptions. Basically, a generic drug is simply a copy of a brand-name drug that is the same with regard to dosage, strength, and efficacy as the brand-name product. Generic drugs are often created when the patents of brand-name drugs expire, allowing them to be produced by companies other than the original manufacturer. All generic drugs (unlike food supplements or so-called "natural" drugs) must also be approved by the FDA, so they should be as safe to take as brand-name drugs.

In general, generic drugs are less expensive than brand-name drugs, because the manufacturers of generic drugs have not had to bear the same costs of development and marketing as the original manufacturer. Because they are less expensive, some company health plans or insurance carriers require that their employees or clients use generic drugs whenever possible. Occasionally, a pharmacy will automatically substitute a generic drug, or at least ask you if you'd prefer the generic equivalent of a drug that your doctor prescribed. Although generic drugs are usually identical to the original brand-name product, differences in formulation can occur. It is always a good idea to ask your doctor whether or not you should consider the generic version of the prescribed drug.

MEDICATIONS USED IN THE TREATMENT OF SINUSITIS AND RHINITIS

An Up-to-Date Guide to Over-the-Counter and Prescription Medicines

Analgesics

Analgesics are products that are designed to reduce mild pain and fever. Such products are often recommended for those suffering from sinus headaches or pain in the jaw or face caused by the swelling resulting from sinus congestion or infection. Aspirin is probably the most common of all analgesics. Originally compounded from willow bark, it was introduced to the market in 1899. It is now used to relieve pain in many areas of the body as well as taken to prevent heart problems. Aspirin is contraindicated for those with Samter's or ASA Triad. Stomach pain is a common side effect of aspirin.

Other more recently introduced analgesics include ibuprofen (Advil® and Motrin®), naproxen (Aleve® and Naprosyn®) and acetominophen (Tylenol®). Together with aspirin, these drugs are referred to as nonsteroidal anti-inflammatory drugs (NSAIDs) because, unlike steroids, they don't treat inflammation by suppressing the immune system. NSAIDs relieve pain by inhibiting the enzyme cyclooxygenase that produces hormone-like substances called prostaglandins which, in turn, cause pain and inflammation. The products mentioned above are available either over-the-counter or by prescription (e.g. ibuprofen). None of these analgesics, with the exception of acetaminophen (Tylenol®) and the COX-2 inhibitors, should be taken by individuals with Samter's Triad; otherwise, a potentially fatal anaphylactic reaction can occur. Drugs of the COX-2 class are available by prescription and include Celebrex® and Vioxx®, drugs usually prescribed to treat the pain associated with arthritis.

Antibiotics

Antibiotics are part of a group of medications known as anti-infectives because they are derived from bacteria and are used to treat bacterial infections. Because rhinosinusitis is frequently caused by a bacterial infection, antibiotics are often the first choice of medication, particularly in patients with acute sinusitis. Relief from symptoms is generally experienced within a few days, and symptoms disappear within two weeks of beginning antibiotic therapy. Unfortunately, antibiotics may be less effective in treating recurrent or chronic sinusitis than acute sinusitis. This is because many strains of bacteria are resistant to antibiotics and because, although a bacterial infection may worsen the symptoms of chronic rhinosinusitis, as noted previously, the infection is probably not the underlying cause of the problem. When resistance occurs, the doctor may prescribe another type of antibiotic or recommend another treatment such as surgery. It should also be noted that antibiotics require a prescription.

Antibiotics are part of a group of medications known as anti-infectives because they are derived from bacteria and are used to treat bacterial infections such as sinusitis.

As we discussed earlier, some antibiotics are considered "broad spectrum" because they are used to treat a wide variety of different types of bacterial infections. Others are considered "narrow spectrum" because they are prescribed to treat a specific type of bacteria.

Penicillins are the oldest type of antibiotics and are similar in structure to cephalosporins. These two types of antibiotics work by actually killing bacteria rather than inhibiting bacterial growth. Penicillins are available as capsules, tablets, liquids, and injections. Dosage and method of administration vary, depending on the nature of the infection. Amoxicillin-clavulanate (Augmentin) is one of the most frequently recommended antibiotics for the treatment of sinusitis. The most common side effects are diarrhea and rashes. Unfortunately, many people are allergic to penicillin.

PENICILLINS

BRAND NAME	MANUFACTURER	GENERIC NAME
Amoxil	GlaxoSmithKline	amoxicillin
Augmentin	GlaxoSmithKline	amoxicillin clavulanate potassium
Unasyn	Pfizer	ampicillin sodium

CEPHALOSPORINS. Cephalosporins, like penicillins, are broad spectrum antibiotics that kill many types of bacteria. Like penicillins, cephalosporins vary in dosage depending on the nature of the infection. The most common side effects are diarrhea and skin rashes. If you are allergic to any cephalosporins or penicillin, you should check with your doctor before taking these antibiotics. Also, they should never be combined with alcohol. Cephalosporins have the advantage over penicillins in that they tend to cause fewer allergic reactions and generally are considered broader spectrum antibiotics than penicillins. They may also cause fewer gastrointestinal side effects. However, they are usually more expensive than penicillins.

CEPHALOSPORINS

Brand Name	Manufacturer	Generic Name
Cedax®	Blovail	ceftibuten dihydrate
Ceftin®	GlaxoSmithKline	cefuroxime axetil
Duricef®	Warner Chilcott	cefadroxil
Keflex Pulvules®	Eli Lilly & Co.	cephalexin
Lorabid®	Pfizer	loracarbef
Omnicef®	Abbott	cefdinir
Suprax®	Wyeth	cefixime
Spectracef®	TAP Pharmaceuticals	cefditoren
Vantin®	Pharmacia & Upjohn	cefpodoxime proxetil

QUINOLONES AND FLUROQUINOLONES. Quinolones and fluro-quinolones are synthetic antibacterial medications. They are generally administered orally, but are available in intravenous form for particularly serious infections. It appears that bacteria can readily and quickly acquire resistance to many of the quinolones. They are therefore generally reserved for infections in which other antibiotics have failed, or for situations in which a culture and sensitivity have demonstrated that they are the best antibiotic. In general, they have a low incidence of gastrointestinal upset, but may cause some other side effects such as dizziness and some temporary weakness of the tendons. Accordingly, heavy exercise should be avoided when taking the quinolone antibiotics, particularly if they are also being taken with a course of oral steroids. Additionally, as a class, the quinolone antibiotics tend to increase sun sensitivity.

QUINOLONES AND FLUOROQUINOLONES

Brand Name	Manufacturer	Generic Name
Avelox®	Bayer	moxifloxacin hydrochloride
Cipro®	Bayer	ciprofloxacin
Tequin®	Bristol Meyers Squibb	gatifloxacin
Levaquin®	Ortho-McNeil	levofloxacin

MACROLIDES. Macrolides are a class of antibiotics that work by inhibiting bacterial protein synthesis. Macrolides include erythromycin, clarithromycin, and azithromycin. Interestingly, research has demonstrated that macrolide antibiotics also have some general anti-inflammatory and antibacterial actions and therefore, unlike other antibiotics, may be of benefit even in a situation where the actual bacteria present are not sensitive to them.

MACROLIDES

Brand Name	Manufacturer	Generic Name
Biaxin®	Abbott	clarithromycin
Zithromax®	Pfizer	azithromycin

KETOLIDES. Ketolides are a new class of macrolides that have been developed to combat bacteria that have become resistant to macrolides. Telithromycin, marketed as Ketek® by its manufacturer, Aventis, is the only ketolide currently on the market.

TETRACYCLINES. Tetracyclines are classified as broad spectrum antibiotics because they can be used to treat a wide variety of infections. Tetracyclines are available as capsules, tablets, liquids, or injections. Generally, tetracyclines work best when taken on an empty stomach with a full glass of water. However, doxycycline is a tetracycline derivative that is not significantly affected by milk or milk products, and taking it with milk may help to reduce gastric irritation. Like a number of other antibiotics, tetracylines should not be taken in pregnancy, and in childhood they can cause tooth discoloration if taken before the permanent teeth have come in. Those patients taking tetracyclines should also avoid exposure to the sun. Doxycycline (Vibramycin®), manufactured by Pfizer, should be taken with adequate fluids to ensure that it does not remain in the esophagus, where it can cause significant irritation.

TOPICAL ANTIBIOTIC SOLUTIONS AND NEBULIZED ANTIBIOTICS. An antibiotic can be added to a saline irrigation in a situation in which superficial infection or recurrent infections are present.

These solutions can then be used as a nasal irrigation, spray, or nebulized solution.

All of the antibiotic solutions and all of the methods of instillation have their proponents. However, at present, none of these methodologies has been proven superior to another, and the concept of adding an antibiotic, although intuitively reasonable, has not been proven superior to the use of saline solution alone.

A nebulized antibiotic solution is an antibiotic in the form of very small droplets of liquid that are inhaled (similar in principle to a cold steam humidifier). Nebulized antibiotics are generally applied for ten to fifteen minutes twice a day for two to three weeks. The supposed advantage of nebulized antibiotics is that the antibiotic makes direct contact with the site of the infection. Moreover, there is concern that nebulized antibiotics are primarily deposited in the very front of the nose around the nostril and that all of the antibiotic solutions might add to the problem of antibiotic resistance. However, when a patient continues to have recurrent infections following surgery (when all the sinuses have been completely opened up), the use of a topical antibiotic is a reasonable consideration.

Generally, whether the antibiotic solutions are mixed by the patient or by a pharmacy, the solutions should never be kept for more than one week in the refrigerator, because opening the sterile saline solution to add the antibiotic creates the potential for contamination (unless it is done in a sterile manufacturing environment). Additionally, the long-term stability of the antibiotic in many of these solutions is not known.

NEBULIZED ANTIBIOTICS

BRAND NAME	MANUFACTURER	GENERIC NAME
Bactroban®	GlaxoSmithKline	mupirocin calcium
Fortaz®	GlaxoSmithKline	ceftazidime sodium

Corticosteroids

Corticosteroids are powerful anti-inflammatory agents. Unlike antibiotics, they do not fight infections. However, they do play an important part in treating chronic rhinosinusitis because this disease has a significant inflammatory element. Indeed, the inflammatory aspect of chronic rhinosinusitis appears to have a greater effect than underlying bacterial component.

Topical Nasal Steroids

Topical steroids are those that are applied directly to a specific area of the body, such as the nose. They suppress the body's inflammatory response, that is, the body's ability to cause swelling specifically in the area to which they are applied. Nasal corticosteroids are an essentially safe form of steroids and are currently recommended as the first line of treatment of allergic rhinitis. There is also evidence that they are of benefit in chronic rhinosinusitis, if used on a regular basis, as well as in the treatment of asthma.

The benefits provided by corticosteroids are:
1. Reduction of inflammation in the sinuses.
2. Reduction of the reactivity of the nasal mucosa.
3. Enabling treatment of the allergic component of allergic fungal sinusitis following surgery.
4. Help to shrink polyps.
5. Helping to control Samter's Triad (ASA Triad), the combination of polyps, asthma, and sensitivity to aspirin.

Nasal corticosteroids are prescription products, and are often combined with a course of antibiotics to treat chronic rhinosinusitis. They are typically sprayed or inhaled once or twice a day. Dosages vary, depending on the age of the patient and the severity of the discomfort. The most common side effects of topical nasal steroids are nasal irritation and occasional bleeding, particularly during the winter when the air is dry. Reducing the dosage usually controls these side effects.

It is also helpful, when the tip of the spray bottle is in the nose, to slightly angle it outward on each side (toward the eye), so that the spray does not all land on the nasal septum and irritate it. Some sprays may cause discomfort and patients may occasionally get headaches associated with the use of nasal sprays. However, generally the side effects are mild, even with regular long-term usage. Although topical steroids are generally safe, even for very long-term use, there is some evidence that, over a period of several years, they may somewhat increase the risk of glaucoma and can contribute to osteoporosis. However, used as prescribed, the benefits of long-term use vastly outweigh potential risks. Listed below are some commonly prescribed corticosteroid nasal sprays.

Corticosteroid Nasal Sprays

Brand Name	Manufacturer	Generic Name
Beconase® Vancenase®	GlaxoSmithKline	beclomethasone dipropionte
Flonase®	GlaxoSmithKline	fluticasone propionate
Nasalide®	Elan	flunisolide
Nasarel®	Elan	flunisolide
Nasacort®, Tri-Nasal®	Aventis	triamcinolone acetonide
Nasonex®	Schering Plough	mometasone furoate monohydrate
Rhinocort®	AstraZeneca	budesonide

Oral Steroids

Oral steroids are ingested or taken as tablets. These steroids, such as Medrol® and Prednisone®, are powerful anti-inflammatory agents that are very effective in reducing the underlying inflammation in both chronic rhinosinusitis and asthma. In severe asthma, they can be lifesaving, and in chronic rhinosinusitis they can make an enormous difference in disease control because they are significantly more effective than the topical steroids. Unfortunately, they can also have potentially serious side effects and are therefore usually reserved for situations where topical steroids are ineffective.

In both sinusitis and asthma, one type of blood cell (the eosinophil) becomes attracted to the area of inflammation and further enhances the inflammation by releasing some toxic compounds at the site of the inflammation. Steroids decrease the recruitment of eosinophils and also help to stabilize them so that they are less likely to release their toxic compounds. Additionally, they decrease the swelling (edema) of the tissue and, as a result, increase clearance of mucus by the cilia, enabling the mucosa to better clear bacteria and fungi, and helping to further reduce inflammation. Thus, steroids are very effective in treating the underlying causes of rhinosinusitis.

Unfortunately, steroids taken by mouth also have frequent and significant side effects, particularly if their dosage is not carefully managed. When taken orally or by injection, they can cause irritability and insomnia and, particularly at higher doses, raise the blood pressure, blood sugar, and cholesterol, cause hyperacidity and indigestion, and raise the pressure in the eye. They cause some fluid retention, increased appetite, and weight gain. These changes are reversible when the steroids are discontinued; however, there may be some feeling of depression when the steroids are tapered or stopped. The longer-term use of oral steroids also tends to reduce our own body's production of these hormones, so that we do not have the same ability to react with increased production at times of infection or stress.

The most serious side effect is that a small percentage of people will develop serious damage to a joint or joints (avascular necrosis), a disorder that also sometimes occurs in people who do not take steroids. The risk of avascular necrosis as a side effect of steroid use is greatly enhanced by smoking and/or drinking alcohol and, when it occurs, replacement of affected joint or joints is frequently required.

Additionally, over time, steroid use will increase the likelihood of osteoporosis or cataracts. When someone is on long-term oral steroid therapy, it is important that they take supplemental calcium (1000 - 1500 mg) and vitamin D (400 – 800 IU) on a daily basis to help to avoid problems with osteoporosis. We usually recommend a bone density study six months into the treatment, and every one to two years thereafter, as well as an annual eye examination by an ophthalmologist.

Generally, oral steroids should be prescribed in the lowest possible dose necessary to treat the problem. It is very important not to miss doses and to take the medication as prescribed. The dose is usually tapered down before it is stopped—indeed, tapering down the dose is critical if it has been used long-term. It is vital to take oral steroids exactly as prescribed. Used carefully, oral steroids are an extremely important part of the management of both severe chronic rhinosinusitis and asthma, but their dosage must be carefully managed.

Finally, because long-term steroids suppress our own ability to respond to stress, someone who is currently on long-term oral steroid therapy, or who has been on long-term oral steroid therapy in the past six months or so, may need to take additional steroids by mouth if they develop a significant infection, are in a serious accident, or have surgery.

You should inform anyone treating you if you have been on long term oral steroid therapy. Some people who are on long-term steroids are also advised to wear a warning bracelet in the event that they may need medical treatment and are unable to explain to the attending medical personnel that they are taking steroids.

Anti-Inflammatory Medications

Cromolyn sodium is an anti-inflammatory medicine that prevents the mucous membranes or the airways from swelling when they are exposed to an allergy trigger. Therefore, it is different from over-the-counter antibiotic nasal sprays. Cromolyn is available as a metered dose inhaler liquid that can be used in a nebulizer, and as a powder-filled capsule that can be inhaled by using a dry powder inhaler. It is not a decongestant, and is not helpful in treating the common cold. However, it blocks the allergic reaction in the nose and can be very helpful for someone with significant nasal allergies. To be continuously effective, however, it must be used four to six times a day, which is difficult for anyone to do.

Accordingly, we typically recommend it for specific allergic reactions, rather than to be used all the time. For instance, it is helpful for a person with nasal grass allergies, who wants to cut the grass or play a round of golf. In such a situation, use of cromolyn about 20 minutes prior to the exposure will significantly block the nasal reaction, reducing sneezing, congestion, and runny nose. The only common side effect is a dry cough. Nasalcrom® is the most common brand name for nasal cromolyn sodium, but other preparations are available for use (Cromlom®, Intal®, and Opticom®).

Decongestants

Decongestants reduce the amount of swelling or congestion of the lining of the nose by reducing the blood flow, thereby increasing the size of the nasal passages. They thus relieve pressure produced by swollen, expanded, or dilated blood vessels in the membranes of the nose and air passages. They do not, however, relieve runny noses or treat inflammation, which is generally caused by a bacterial, fungal, or viral infection. Two types of decongestants are available, those used as a topical spray and those taken orally by mouth. Both are widely available as over-the-counter medications.

Topical decongestant sprays should be administered one nostril at a time. Because those with rhinosinusitis may have an infection that might be contagious, nasal sprays or droppers should not be shared with another person. These sprays are very effective but should not be used for more than three to five days; if used on a long-term basis, they can cause a gradual worsening of the condition they are designed to treat, as well as an increasing dependency as a result of a rebound effect. As with other medicine dependencies, topical decongestant dependency may develop slowly, and have minimal side effects initially, but the long-term effect on the nose can be dramatic.

Oral decongestants, such as Sudafed®, are less effective and may also cause systemic side effects (that is, affecting more than just the nose), but are safer for long-term use. The chemicals in decongestants are related to adrenaline—a stimulant produced naturally in the body—so, some people get a jittery feeling or interference with sleep as a side effect. Because diet pills also contain stimulants, anyone taking diet pills should avoid decongestants.

Decongestants constrict blood vessels and can increase blood pressure. Accordingly, they should not be taken by anyone with a history of high blood pressure, heart disease, or glaucoma. They are also not advised for men with prostrate problems as they can aggravate this condition.

Long-acting Over-the-Counter Decongestant Sprays (6-12 hours)

Brand Name	Manufacturer	Generic Name
Afrin®	Schering Plough	oxymetazoline HCL
Dristan 12-Hour®	Wyeth	oxymetazoline HCL
Neo-Synephrine 12-Hour®	Bayer	oxymetazoline HCL
Sudafed®	Pfizer	pseudoephedrine HCL
Vicks Sinex®	Procter & Gamble	oxymetazoline HCL

Short Acting Decongestants (4 hours)

Brand Name	Manufacturer	Generic Name
Dristan Mist Spray®	Wyeth	phenylephrine HCL
Naphcon A®	Alcon	naphazoline HCL
Neo-Synephrine®	Bayer	phenylephrine HCL
Privine®	Heritage	naphazoline HCL
Vicks Sinex®	Procter & Gamble	phenylephrine HCL

Oral Antihistamines

Antihistamines are medications that block the effects of histamine, one of the chemicals released in an allergic reaction. Because of this they are helpful to patients with allergic rhinitis, and they may also have some effect in blocking some of the reactions in chronic rhino-sinusitis. Unfortunately, they sometimes also thicken and dry the mucus, and this can make it more difficult for the cilia to clear. If this happens to you, you should discuss with your doctor whether you should continue or stop the use of them.

Antihistamines are often taken on a regular basis during allergy season by people with seasonal allergies. They are often cheaper than topical nasal steroid sprays and have the benefit of reducing the allergic reaction in the eyes, which a topical nasal steroid cannot do.

On the other hand, they are often less effective than topical nasal steroids in the reduction of nasal symptoms and drowsiness is a common side effect. Usually, drowsiness is just a nuisance but, when someone is driving or operating heavy machinery, it can be very dangerous. Additionally, antihistamines markedly increase the effects of alcohol and further reduce a person's ability to drive or operate heavy machinery. Antihistamines can also cause dry eyes or mouth and can be a problem for people with an enlarged prostate.

In the past 10 to 15 years, a number of less sedating antihistamines have been introduced to the market. Because sedation is helpful in reducing some of the allergic symptoms, for some people these so-called non-sedating antihistamines may not be as effective as the older antihistamines. Additionally, most of these newer antihistamines are only available by prescription (for example, Allegra®, Zyrtec®, and Clarinex®). However, in 2003 the very popular Claritin® was made available as an over-the-counter medication.

OVER-THE-COUNTER ORAL ANTIHISTAMINES AND ORAL DECONGESTANT COMBINATIONS

BRAND NAME	MANUFACTURER	GENERIC NAME
Actifed®	Pfizer	Triprolidine HCL and pseudoephedrine HCL
Benadryl®	Pfizer	Diphenhydramine citrate
Claritin®	Schering Plough	loratadine
Contac®	GlaxoSmithKline	acetaminophen
Chlor-Trimeton®	Schering Plough	chlorpheniramine maleate
Dimetapp®	Wyeth	phenylpropanolamine
Drixoral®	Schering Plough	dexbrompheniramine and pseudoephedrine

PRESCRIPTION ORAL ANTIHISTAMINES

BRAND NAME	MANUFACTURER	GENERIC NAME
Allegra®	Aventis	fexofenadine HCL
Clarinex®	Schering Plough	desloratadine
Zyrtec®	Pfizer	cetirizine HCL

Antihistamines are also sold as antihistamine and decongestant combinations (for example, Allegra D, Claritin D). These combinations add the effect of a decongestant and, because the decongestant also has a slight stimulation effect, the sedation in the antihistamine may be somewhat less noticeable. However, because decongestants do have a tendency to raise blood pressure, they may be less ideal for long-term use.

Mucolytics and Expectorants

Mucolytics are drugs that are designed to help promote sinus drainage by thinning mucus. Expectorants are designed to thin mucus in the chest, which allows it to be coughed up from the lungs. Their efficacy is variable, but they are safe and can be helpful in some people. If you have chronic rhinosinusitis, it is worth trying them to see if they provide some relief. Some mucolytics are combined with decongestants and, as with antihistamine-decongestant combinations, are probably best not used long term because of the potential effect on blood pressure. All mucolytic agents may increase fertility in women of childbearing age by thinning cervical mucus and enhancing transport across the cervix. There are dozens of expectorant products available today.

EXPECTORANTS AND MUCOLYTICS

BRAND NAME	MANUFACTURER	GENERIC NAME
Breonesin®	Sanofi Winthrop	guaifenesin
DuroTuss®	3M Pharmaceuticals	pseudoephdrine, hydrocodone, guaifenesin
Glytuss®	Merz	guaifenesin
Humibid, L.A.®	Adams Laboratories	guaifenesin
Robitussin®	Wyeth	guaifenesin

Leukotriene Antagonists

Leukotriene antagonists are oral drugs that block leukotrienes, another class of inflammatory agents released in allergies, and some kinds of inflammation. Leukotreine antagonists are very helpful in the management of asthma, but do not appear to be as effective in the management of either chronic rhinosinusitis or nasal polyps. However, they have significantly fewer side effects than oral steroids and may be worth trying, even in the absence of asthma.

LEUKOTRIENE ANTAGONISTS

BRAND NAME	MANUFACTURER	GENERIC NAME
Accolate®	AstraZeneca	zafirlukast
Singulair®	Merck	montelukast

Anti-IgE Antibodies

Xolair® (omalizumab) is one of a very new class of medications, an antibody made to directly block immunoglobulin E (IgE), the primary antibody implicated in allergic and asthmatic reactions. It is extremely expensive and can only be administered by injection every two to four weeks. However, it has been proven very effective in preventing asthma attacks in patients with severe asthma that has not responded well to other medications. At present, it is only approved for use in severe asthma. However, it is possible that it may also have some effect in severe rhinosinusitis that is not responding to currently approved medications.

What if Medication Does Not Provide Relief from Symptoms?

Chronic rhinosinusitis can be a stubborn condition and, despite our best efforts, sometimes symptoms continue. Unfortunately, for some people, their rhinosinusitis will remain incurable by medication. For these people, often the best option will be to consider surgery. In the next chapter we will discuss what surgical options are now available.

13

FUNCTIONAL ENDOSCOPIC SINUS SURGERY

What to Expect from Surgery

SURGERY FOR SINUSITIS USED TO BE A VERY unpleasant option frequently involving external incisions, significant discomfort, and a high failure rate. However, approximately 20 years ago, sinus imaging improved, and endoscopes became more available for diagnosis. This improved visualization enabled me, along with some physicians in Europe, to recognize that some of the established concepts about the role of specific sinuses in rhinosinusitis were not correct.

With improved endoscopic visualization and radiographic imaging, the importance of the ethmoid sinuses and the ostiomeatal complex became evident as key areas in the development of inflammation. We could now identify, both endoscopically and with imaging, how chronic inflammation and obstruction in these areas affected the larger sinuses, such as the maxillary and the frontal sinuses. As a result of these observations, I introduced a technique in the United States that I termed functional endoscopic sinus surgery (FESS). The keystone of the technique was the concept of accurate endoscopic and imaging diagnosis of the key site of disease and the recognition that it was not necessary or desirable to strip the linings from the major sinuses as had been done in the past.

Not surprisingly, at that time these concepts created some controversy with surgeons more familiar with the older surgical techniques. Discussions at meetings where I presented the concepts of FESS were often heated and sometimes unpleasant. Even in the usually staid medical literature I was called a "nasal astronomer," and it was said that my statements regarding these techniques were a "presumptuous banality." Nonetheless, over time, these techniques became widely accepted. Studies repeatedly demonstrated that the results were indeed significantly better than with conventional sinus surgical procedures, patient discomfort was dramatically reduced and, of course, external incisions were not required. As a result, Heinz Stammberger (from Graz, Austria), Jim Zinreich (from Baltimore, Maryland), and I have subsequently had the pleasure of teaching these techniques to thousands of surgeons from all over the world. FESS has now become the standard of care for most cases of chronic rhinosinusitis that do not respond well to nonsurgical medical therapy.

More recently, we have extended our endoscopic sinus surgical techniques so that we can now manage tumors, thyroid eye disease, and even some intracranial problems with similar endoscopic intranasal techniques. We have also refined our surgery for chronic rhinosinusitis. We have learned that it is not only important to keep the lining mucosa in place in the major sinuses, but that it is important to avoid exposing bone in any sinus. We have also learned that we need a more complete removal of the areas of disease than we previously thought, because the bone also becomes involved in the inflammatory process. These changes have led to my own surgeries becoming more meticulous and detailed and, as a result, significantly longer procedures than when we first introduced the technique.

Endoscopic sinus surgery has now become a very common procedure. In fact, it is estimated that between 300,000 and 500,000 sinus

surgeries are performed in the United States each year. This procedure avoids much of the discomfort associated with the older surgical
procedures and, when patients are carefully selected and the surgery
is carefully performed, the success rate for the surgeries is very high.

Unfortunately, there is evidence that this surgery is now being
performed too often. Our original concept was that the ostiomeatal
complex and the ethmoid sinuses were critical areas in the development of chronic sinus disease, but some physicians interpreted this as
meaning that disease in this area was the *underlying* cause of chronic
rhinosinusitis, and that surgery should be the *primary* method of treatment. As we have discussed in the prior chapters, this is not the case.
The underlying causes of rhinosinusitis are multiple and include
environmental, allergic, and probably genetic factors.

The primary method of treating chronic rhinosinusitis should be
medication. Surgery is helpful when the treatments reviewed in
Chapter 10 do not work, if medications fail, or when an anatomical
problem exists that cannot be helped by medical treatment. Surgical
intervention is very helpful only when the inflammation becomes
chronic despite nonsurgical medical therapy, and the inflammation is
aggravating the reaction of the mucosa throughout all the sinuses.

What is Functional Endoscopic Sinus Surgery?

Functional endoscopic sinus surgery (FESS) is a minimally invasive
technique that is designed to remove chronic inflammation in key areas
and correct obstructions in the nose and sinuses. The surgery relies on
careful diagnosis using endoscopes and CT imaging. When we first
introduced FESS in the United States during the early 1980s, we performed the majority of surgical cases under local anesthesia. However,
we now know that to get the best results, we need to be much more
meticulous in our surgical techniques than we were at that time.
Accordingly, the surgery today usually takes longer and is performed
under general anesthesia. However, as pointed out earlier, the primary

treatment remains nonsurgical medical therapy, which needs to be continued postoperatively, although typically much less nonsurgical medical therapy is required once the surgical sites have fully healed.

Following FESS, it is critically important to ensure that the sinus cavities heal well and do not close off with scar tissue, and that any persistent low-level inflammation resolves over time. This typically means a period of close endoscopic follow-up by the surgeon, with adjustment of medications, based not upon residual symptoms (most patients feel much better right away), but upon the resolution of the residual inflammation as seen endoscopically. If performed by a capable and experienced physician, FESS is successful in creating a major improvement in symptoms in more than 90 percent of cases. However, since the underlying causes of chronic sinusitis may still be present, approximately 20 percent of patients may require an additional procedure as the years go by. In addition to being a reflection of how well the surgery and postoperative care was performed, the probability of another surgical sinus procedure is significantly dependent on the extent of the disease at the time of the surgery, the nonsurgical medical therapy, and whether or not you are able to avoid the factors that precipitated the sinusitis in the first place.

WHAT IS THE PURPOSE OF FESS? The purpose of FESS is to remove or correct obstructions and remove areas of persistent inflammation, allowing the sinuses to drain, and letting the patient breathe more freely. It also helps topical medications, such as nasal steroid sprays, to actually get into the sinuses, making it easier to control inflammation in the long term.

In recent years, we have also demonstrated that the thin partitions of bone become inflamed in areas close to the areas of chronic mucosal inflammation. Bone inflammation appears to cause the mucosal inflammation to persist, and responds poorly to medical therapy. FESS allows much of these inflamed bone fragments to be removed, thus helping the inflammation to resolve. In addition to opening up the nose and sinuses, FESS will typically resolve the associated facial pressure and pain as well as the low-grade flulike symptoms that may plague a patient with chronic rhinosinusitis.

WHO BENEFITS MOST FROM FESS? In chronic sinusitis, FESS is typically reserved for people who do not get significantly better with nonsurgical medical therapy. In general, the diagnostic evaluation should still show areas of persistent chronic inflammation even following a careful course of medical therapy, as well as structural deformities in the sinus area to be corrected. FESS is also effective for people who have developed expansile cysts in their sinuses (mucoceles) and people with severe acute sinusitis, which is in danger of developing complications. Complications that might indicate FESS is needed include meningitis, orbital cellulitis (infection that spreads to the area surrounding the eye), infection in the bones of the face, and antibiotic resistance. If the patient also has the complication of nasal obstruction due to a septal deformity, this can be corrected at the same time as well.

FESS is effective in removing nasal polyps, and the same techniques have now been extended for the endoscopic removal of tumors. We have also developed modifications of FESS that have enabled surgeons to correct cerebrospinal fluid (CSF) leaks, which are defects between the brain and nose or sinuses that cause a leak of the fluid from around the brain into the nose, with more than a 90 percent success rate. Performing this type of "skull bone" surgery endoscopically dramatically reduces morbitity and complications when compared to craniotomy.

In children, we would obviously prefer to avoid surgery whenever possible, and usually rhinosinusitis will respond to nonsurgical medical therapy and often resolves completely over time. However, when it persists and is severe despite use of the usual medicines, FESS is a realistic option, and the surgery usually can be more limited than in adults because children have such great healing potential.

Patients who are HIV positive often have problems with chronic rhinosinusitis. Endoscopic sinus surgery has been demonstrated to significantly improve nasal and sinus symptoms for these patients, and may allow the sinuses to return completely to normal.

WHAT ARE THE ADVANTAGES OF ENDOSCOPIC SURGERY? Because endoscopic surgery is a minimally invasive surgery, it has many advantages over traditional surgery. There are no external incisions and the function of the sinuses (producing the mucociliary blanket) is restored. Unlike traditional surgery, there is usually little or no post-operative pain, although the follow-up endoscopies can be uncomfortable. Bleeding is usually minimal, the recovery is faster than with traditional surgery, and the success rate is higher.

WHO SHOULD NOT HAVE THE SURGERY? If a patient is not in danger of developing complications, we would not recommend sinus surgery until a prolonged trial of nonsurgical medical therapy has been tried. This prolonged trial of medical therapy would usually include environmental control and treatment of allergies, if present, the regular use of topical nasal steroid preparations, more than one full antibiotic course (preferably with at least one course selected based on the results of nasal or sinus culture), and possibly a short course of oral steroids.

Endoscopic sinus surgery will not be helpful to someone who has uncontrolled environmental allergies unless the inflammation has become so severe that it is clearly making the allergic reactions much worse. It will also not be helpful if, in the long run, the patient continues to be exposed to the same environmental irritants that caused the problem to develop in the first place.

Smoke from tobacco or marijuana are two of those environmental irritants. For this reason, I do not recommend elective endoscopic sinus surgery for someone who has not yet given up smoking. In fact, one of the primary purposes of the surgery is to open up the sinuses and, if this is performed on a patient who only had mild inflammation and is still exposed to such irritants as tobacco smoke or environmental allergens, there is the potential to make the rhinosinusitis worse by exposing new areas of relatively normal mucosa to the same irritants that initially caused the problem.

How Do I Choose a Surgeon?

Before you undergo any type of surgery, you should try to make sure that your surgeon is both experienced and well-respected in his or her field. Certainly, it is important to ensure that the surgeon is board-certified in otolaryngology, but this alone is probably not sufficient. You should try to talk to people in your area who may have had the same surgeon, keeping in mind that sometimes what the patient primarily experiences is a surgeon's bedside manner, and not his or her surgical skills.

If a magazine in your area publishes a "best doctor" list, this can also be helpful. There are books listing the best doctors in America, which can also serve as a guide for patients who may be willing to travel for surgery. However, none of these lists is definitive, and they do not include many excellent physicians. There are also Internet referral services, but you will need to evaluate whether the service that you use is just paid advertising or whether it really evaluates a surgeon on good data.

As with all surgical procedures, you want a surgeon who performs a significant number of the type of procedure you are going to have performed. At the same time, in the case of endoscopic sinus surgery, you do not want someone who either performs surgery too often (when nonsurgical medical therapy might work), or who does not spend the necessary time and effort postoperatively to ensure that the areas that were operated on are healing optimally.

It is impossible to perform a large volume of endoscopic sinus surgery each week *and* perform the postoperative care required to ensure that each patient heals well and in a timely manner. Although not readily available, probably the most reliable information regarding a surgeon's surgical ability can be obtained from talking to the operating-room nurses at the hospital where the physician practices. These nurses work with a number of physicians and have an excellent basis of knowledge to evaluate surgical abilities. As a result, they typically know more about the surgeon than a referring physician. Although a referral from your internist or family doctor is helpful, it is also worth asking around. Although the surgery itself may seem relatively minor, the potential for either achieving significant improvement, or for causing additional problems which can be difficult to resolve, is considerable.

If you have already had surgery and the problem has either not improved or has recurred, or if you have a very unusual problem, you may want to consider consulting an otolaryngologist who is trained in a subspecialty within the field of rhinology. These specialists have more training and additional skills that help them to deal with the more difficult sinus and nasal problems, and they typically only take care of these specialized problems. Although the number of rhinology specialists is limited nationally, there are now such specialists in the larger cities and at a number of the larger university medical centers.

What Results Should I Expect from Surgery?

In most cases, surgery will not resolve the underlying causes of rhinosinusitis, so some ongoing nonsurgical medical therapy will still be required. However, when patients are carefully selected for surgery, the results from surgery are excellent when combined with ongoing medical therapy and meticulous postoperative care, although the ultimate effect of the procedure is usually dependent on the extent of the inflammation at the time of surgery.

In our studies we have demonstrated that well over 90 percent of patients feel significantly better following FESS, even if they have had prior sinus surgery that failed. We can demonstrate that these patients use fewer medications, and that more than 90 percent of those who have asthma also get improvement in that disorder. Moreover, when combined with appropriate medical therapy, we have documented that these improvements are maintained, even many years after the surgical procedure.

The most dramatic improvements tend to occur in nasal congestion and discomfort, but patients also report significant improvements in their overall health and well-being when the chronic inflammation is controlled, and these improvements have been documented scientifically. Unfortunately, when the sense of smell has been affected by the inflammation preoperatively, however, the long-term 100 percent recovery of the patient's olfactory sense cannot be guaranteed.

Postnasal discharge is the one symptom that sometimes does not get significantly better; it also takes longest to improve. This is not surprising because the surgery opens up the sinuses, and the increased discharge may continue until all the remaining inflammation resolves. Therefore, the problem of postnasal discharge may not improve for months or even years.

HOW DO I PREPARE FOR SURGERY? Preparation for surgery will vary depending on several factors, including your age and any other diseases or complications that you may have. Your surgeon will probably recommend a checkup with your internist or family physician if you are older or have any medical problems that could be an issue with the surgery or the anesthesia. It is important that you let the surgeon know if you take any medications or herbal remedies.

You will typically be asked not to take any aspirin, ginko biloba, or vitamin E for two weeks prior to the surgery, since these are some of the substances that thin the blood and may cause excess bleeding. For the same reason, you should also abstain from taking any medication that contains ibuprofen for at least five days prior to surgery.

It is important to let the surgeon know if you or a close family member have any bleeding tendencies, or have had significant problems from anesthesia. It is also a good idea to remind the surgeon if you have any medication allergies. If you have asthma or marked intranasal inflammation, your surgeon may start you on a course of oral steroids prior to the surgery. This helps to reduce the chances of getting an asthma attack during or after the surgery and reduces the bleeding in the nose.

You will probably also be asked not to eat or drink anything after midnight the night before the surgery. Your surgeon may also ask you not to take any of your regular medications, such as heart medications, on the day of the surgery. Even if your surgeon says it is all right to take them, you may be asked to take them with a minimal amount of water.

WHAT TYPE OF ANESTHETIC IS REQUIRED? Although FESS can be performed using either local or general anesthesia or both, at present we usually perform more of the surgeries under general anesthesia because, as mentioned earlier, we are more meticulous during the surgery and it therefore typically takes longer than it did previously. However, the minor endoscopic surgical procedures can easily be performed under local anesthesia with some intravenous sedation ("twilight sleep"). More extensive surgeries can also be performed in this fashion when this is medically necessary, or when general anesthesia is not advisable. A general anesthetic is used when the surgery is performed on children.

HOW LONG DOES THE SURGERY TAKE? It is difficult to predict exactly how long your surgery will take, since it will depend entirely on the number of sinuses that need to be opened and the severity of the inflammation, as well as on the surgical techniques used. When FESS was first introduced, we performed the surgery more quickly, but we were less meticulous then about removing all the areas of disease and not as careful abut not exposing bone. We now know that it is important to remove the disease completely and to minimize exposure of bone. By performing the surgery so scrupulously, we can also reduce the potential for postoperative scarring and decrease the need for postoperative care. Therefore, the surgery takes significantly longer than before; it usually lasts from about one to three hours and, occasionally, even longer. However, because general anesthesia is so much safer and intra-operative monitoring is much more effective, the length of surgery is not a concern for the patient. As long as the surgery is being performed under general anesthesia, the length of surgery is only important for the surgeon and your family in the waiting room!

HOW IS THE SURGERY PERFORMED? Prior to deciding on surgical intervention, the surgeon will have performed an endoscopic examination and a CT scan to identify the areas of inflammation and obstruction as precisely as possible. (However, typically the inflammation is somewhat more marked and more extensive when the surgery is actually performed than can be accurately diagnosed preoperatively.)

After you are either sedated or asleep, your nose will be numbed with local anesthesia. This reduces both the amount of general anesthetic required and the amount of bleeding. The surgeon then introduces the telescope or endoscope into the nose and, alongside it, different types of instruments for removing tissue. One such instrument is called a microdebrider. This instrument is equipped with a blade and a rotor that can accurately remove the obstruction without damaging the area around it, and also carries a small vacuum cleaner that removes whatever obstruction or diseased tissue that has been removed by the blade and rotor.

Through the use of the endoscope the surgeon gets a close-up, magnified view of the nose, either by looking through the endoscope or by attaching a tiny camera and looking at a video screen. The endoscope enables him to see in great detail the problem areas.

A number of years ago we used lasers for this type of surgery, but we now know that the heat they produce can cause unnecessary damage to the delicate adjacent tissues, and alternative methods of removing the disease are usually preferred.

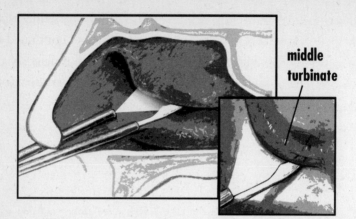

Figure 19. *Functional Endoscopic Sinus Surgery, a minimally invasive technique, removes chronic inflammation in key areas and corrects obstructions in the nose and sinuses. Endoscope and other instruments such as microdebriders are introduced into the nose to accurately remove obstructions without damaging the area around them.*

IS THE SURGERY PAINFUL? FESS should not cause significant pain. Indeed, the vast majority of people undergoing FESS feel dramatically improved in the early postoperative period. However, early improvement in symptoms is not the end point of the management by a good surgeon. By performing regular office endoscopies in the postoperative period, the surgeon will ensure that not only the symptoms improve, but that the remaining inflammation, which may not be causing symptoms at this point in time, resolve. This will help to ensure that problems do not return in the future.

HOW LONG IS THE RECOVERY PERIOD FOLLOWING FESS? If there is extensive sinus involvement, marked nasal polyps, and failed prior surgery, resolution of the residual inflammation can take a long time and can require extensive postoperative medical management. However, even with the most extensive disease, there will be improvement—albeit slowly—over time. When patients with the most severe and extensive chronic sinusitis, asthma, and diffuse nasal polyps ask me what to expect from surgery, I tell them that after one year they will say that they are doing much better; however, they probably will have had several courses of antibiotics and steroids during the year. After two years, they typically say, "It has been my best year yet." At three years, with continued medical management in addition to the surgery, they will usually say that it has totally changed their lives. In extensive disease, the residual inflammation, which often involves the underlying bone, takes a long time before it completely settles down. In more minor disease, the inflammation will settle down within a few days to a few weeks after surgery.

HOW SHOULD I DECIDE IF SURGERY IS RIGHT FOR ME? The most important issue in deciding whether or not to have surgery is how much trouble you are having with the symptoms of sinusitis. In most cases, the chances of serious complications from chronic sinusitis are relatively small and, unlike polyps on the bowel, polyps in the nose are not true tumors and will not become cancerous if they are left in place. So this concern is not a reason to undergo surgery. Generally, however, if left untreated, chronic sinusitis will slowly worsen over time and may cause more problems, with more discomfort and pain as you get older.

It is important to realize that the surgery is not a "silver bullet." Although the chances of getting a very marked improvement in symptoms is excellent, it is probable that you will still have to take some medications after surgery and that all your symptoms will not be resolved completely, at least in the early postoperative period. Although there are some potentially serious complications from sinus surgery, the frequency with which these complications occurs is very low when the surgery is performed by a skilled surgeon, and fear of these rare but serious complications is therefore not usually a sufficient reason to avoid surgery. Of course, if you do have a tumor or a complication caused by sinusitis, the surgery is more mandatory, and the surgeon may strongly recommend early surgery.

WHAT ARE THE RISKS AND COMPLICATIONS OF ENDOSCOPIC SINUS SURGERY? Every medical procedure involves some risk, however small. As with all surgeries, there is always some chance that the patient may have an adverse reaction to the anesthetic. However, the primary risk of FESS is that it may not resolve all the symptoms and, if not properly performed, or if a bad postoperative infection occurs, it could actually make your symptoms worse. Because the surgery occurs in an area where infection is often present, there is always the possibility of postoperative infection, despite the fact that most doctors will prescribe an antibiotic following sinus surgery. In any case, for the reasons outlined previously, it is expected that, following this type of surgery, the residual inflammation will take some time to resolve and, in very extensive disease, it could take a long time.

Bleeding during the surgery is usually only a problem for the surgeon, because it makes endoscopic surgery more difficult. It is rarely a problem for the patient and almost never is it sufficient to need a blood transfusion. However, it always is possible that you might have serious bleeding either during or following the surgery.

The sense of smell is typically impaired immediately after FESS, when the lining is swollen, but there is a reasonable probability of it improving (even more than before the surgery) with appropriate postoperative medical therapy. There is, however, also a small chance that, after the surgery, the sense of smell might decrease in the longer term, or it might disappear altogether. In most cases, this would not be a direct effect of the surgery but rather because the surgery has led to inflammation in the olfactory area. Unfortunately, whether the sense of smell returns or not varies, is difficult to guarantee, and is dependent on many pre- and postoperative factors.

There are two components to the decreased sense of smell associated with chronic rhinosinutis. Initially, in chronic sinusitis the loss of sense of smell is usually due to thickening of the lining of the nose. This thickened inflamed lining prevents odors from reaching the olfactory nerve endings, but typically will improve, at least temporarily, with oral steroids or surgery. However, over time, the olfactory nerve itself deteriorates as a result of the chronic inflammation, and this loss appears irreversible. Surgery will typically decrease the swelling of the lining and, if the loss is due to swelling, the sense of smell and taste should improve. However, surgery will not help the sense of smell if the olfactory nerve has become damaged.

The brain and intracranial cavity are above the sinuses, and the eyes on either side of them. Although damage to either of these structures is very rare, the potential complications are very serious. Fortunately, in skilled surgical hands, the potential of risk to these structures is very low, although not completely absent. Accordingly, although you need to be aware of these risks, if you have chosen a skilled and experienced surgeon, damage to either of these structures occurs so rarely that it is not a major factor in whether or not the surgery should be performed.

The sinuses are separated from the intracranial cavity and brain by thin bone, and there is a small chance that this bone could become cracked, or that a small portion could be removed during the surgery. In some situations, inflammation or a tumor will also erode this bone so that is no longer present. If this area is manipulated, there is a risk of creating an opening between the intracranial cavity and the nose. The immediate effect of this crack is a leak of cerebrospinal fluid (CSF) into the nose. The incidence of CSF leak during FESS is from 0.1 to 1 percent, varying somewhat based upon the extent of the surgery being performed and the experience of the surgeon. In surgery to remove tumors or in complicated frontal sinus surgery, the incidence is higher, and in some tumor surgery it may be necessary to deliberately create a CSF leak to remove all of the tumor. A CSF leak itself is not a huge problem as long as it is recognized and closed at the time of the surgery. It would probably only cause you to stay in the hospital for a few extra days and limit your activity somewhat in the postoperative period. However, while it is present, it also creates a pathway for infection to spread intracranially, potentially leading to meningitis or a brain abscess and, if it is not recognized, additional intracranial damage could occur. Therefore, the complications of CSF leak, although much less common than a CSF leak itself, could potentially be life-threatening.

The eyes are also separated from the sinuses by thin bone, and there is a small risk (smaller than the risk of CSF leak) of causing damage to the eye muscles or to the vision. Damage to the eye muscles would cause double vision when both eyes are open. In some cases, but not all, this can be corrected with further surgery. Damage to the eye itself could cause a loss of vision, but this is even more rare. Loss of vision would most likely be caused if the surgery caused bleeding into the eye socket (orbit), which put pressure on the optic nerve. Should such bleeding occur, your doctor would take steps to relieve any pressure on the eye, but there is still some chance of vision loss. There are also some risks associated with anesthesia, although in general these risks have been significantly reduced in recent years.

Although some of these risks are pretty scary, the frequency with which they occur is so low that they are really not major factors in whether or not to have surgery. The real questions are "How much trouble am I having?" and "How much will the surgery help me, since it likely will not take all of my problems away?" The potential complications are also reasons for selecting a surgeon who is skilled and has a good reputation for positive results in sinus surgery.

HOW WILL I FEEL AFTER SURGERY? There is usually little pain after FESS. Unlike the past, we do not pack the nose tightly, so it is usually still possible to breathe through the nose, even in the immediate postoperative period. Still, it is not uncommon to feel somewhat nauseated from the anesthetic and, most likely, you will feel tired.

Some people find that it takes several days or even a week or two before their full energy level returns. Although there is usually no facial bruising or facial swelling, some bruising around the eye can occasionally occur.

Because the nose is not tightly packed, it is normal to have some bloody nasal discharge and to have some nosebleed immediately after the surgery and, from time to time, over the first few days. Later, after a few weeks, there may be a thick brown discharge (a mixture of old blood and mucus) when you blow your nose. This is a sign that the normal mucociliary clearance is becoming reestablished. Some surgeons may recommend that you spend the night after the surgery in the hospital, but for most surgery in which there are no other serious medical conditions, it can be performed on an outpatient basis.

You should avoid bending down or blowing your nose for a few days after the surgery, and refrain from heavy lifting, straining, and rigorous exercise for a couple of weeks. Taking walks and light exercise may be continued, even during the early postoperative period. We recommend that you do not swim for about six weeks after the surgery (because of the risk of infection), but we allow patients to take a trip in an airplane a day or so after the surgery has been performed.

WHAT POSTSURGICAL CARE IS RECOMMENDED? After the surgery has been performed, the patient is usually advised to use a sterile saline (saltwater) spray to reduce the crusting in the nose. Some surgeons will prescribe a saline wash, because this is even more effective at removing crust, but it does carry some risk of introducing infection. Most physicians will prescribe an antibiotic for several weeks and, with cases of more severe inflammation or when you also have asthma, the doctor will probably prescribe a tapering dose of oral steroids. Topical nasal steroids are also usually restarted a few days after the surgery. If you have significant allergies, an antihistamine may also be prescribed.

WHAT POSTOPERATIVE FOLLOW-UP IS REQUIRED? The extent to which your surgeon will follow up with you endoscopically will vary from surgeon to surgeon. Some feel that oral antibiotics and nasal irrigations will allow maximum healing, and will only perform a minimum of endoscopic follow-ups. I, and a number of other surgeons, feel that close endoscopic follow-up is essential because we cannot rely on the patient's symptoms to ensure that the site of surgery is healing well, or to be sure that all the sinuses that we have opened are staying open. Remember that most patients feel better after the surgery, but we want more than an improvement in symptoms; we want to try to ensure that you do not have further sinus problems in the future.

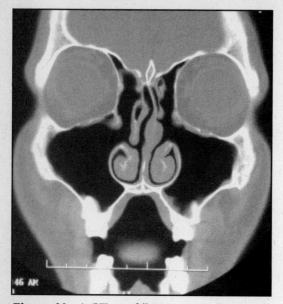

Figure 20. *A CT scan following surgery demonstrates widely open sinuses connecting with the nose. Most postoperative follow up is performed endoscopically because it is now possible to clearly see into the sinuses.*

Typically, I will see the patient the day after surgery, take out the sponges after anesthetizing the nose with a spray, and suction any blood out of the nose and sinuses. I then like to reexamine the nose on a weekly basis until the cavity has healed, using my endoscopic findings to adjust medications, take cultures when necessary, and remove any scar tissue that is starting to form. When the patient is from out of state, these follow-up visits are usually shared with an otolaryngologist who lives in the patient's area.

How long the cavity takes to heal is very dependent on the amount of inflammation present. In minor disease it may be healed in three weeks. In severe disease, particularly when the patient has had one or more prior surgeries and prolonged problems, it can take many months. In this situation, the endoscopic examinations are performed with decreasing frequency after the initial healing phase.

Prior to each of these follow-up examinations, it is recommended that the patient take some pain medication because, although the nose is anesthetized, there can be some discomfort. Your physician will carefully examine the healing in each area that was opened and, if scar tissue is starting to form, will remove it. Your doctor will also look for persistent inflammation and treat it, while trying to ensure that the nasal function is returning to normal.

14

OTHER SURGERIES OF THE SINUSES, HEAD, AND THROAT

A Discussion of Other Surgical Options

Image-Guided Surgery

Everyone's sinus anatomy is different; indeed, it is probably just as different as fingerprints, because they all develop in individual ways. Additionally, both the eyes and the brain are close to the area of surgery. To try to help the surgeon and to reduce the risks of surgery, we have been working for a number of years with different devices that enable physicians to see exactly where the instruments are at any point during the surgery, using the preoperative CT scan or MR scan as guide. This type of surgery is called image-guided surgery, or computer-assisted surgical navigation.

In this type of surgery, the preoperative CT scan is loaded into a computer in the operating room and, after the patient's head position

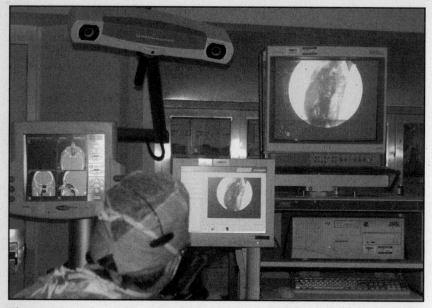

Figure 21: *Using a pre-operative CT or MR scan as a guide, the surgeon can track the progress of a computer guided surgery in three dimensions. With computer guided surgery the surgeon can see where the instruments are both by endoscopic visualization and on the CT scan.*

has also been registered into the computer, different instruments can be tracked by the computer and viewed, superimposed on the CT scan on a video screen during the surgery. Depending on the device, the tracking may be performed by infrared light, optical cameras, or electromagnetic transmitters. As a result, the surgeon is made aware of where the instrument is at any time during the surgery.

When we first started working with these devices about 15 years ago, they were difficult to use and not very accurate. Now they have become easier to use, more available, and more precise. By providing the surgeon with CT pictures in three planes—horizontal (axial); vertical (coronal); and longitudinal (sagittal)—they help the surgeon create a three-dimensional conceptualization of the anatomy and make the surgery less difficult and more complete. Unfortunately, at this time, the accuracy is still not sufficient to ensure that the risk of complications (which is already low) has been further reduced.

Conventional Open Surgery of the Sinus

In some cases, particularly those that are especially severe and for the removal of certain tumors, it may not be possible to use endoscopic surgery. In such cases, it may be necessary to use a more conventional approach. This type of surgery is called open surgery because, unlike endoscopic surgery, it requires that an incision be made through a location in the mouth, in the forehead, or on the face. Such a procedure can be quite effective, but it may also leave some scarring, result in a longer recuperation, and be more painful than endoscopic surgery.

Caldwell-Luc Operation

This surgery was originally designed to clear infection and to improve drainage of the maxillary sinuses. It is almost never performed today to treat infection because the results with endoscopic sinus surgery are usually better. However, it may be necessary for tumors, or in some other unusual situations.

The Caldwell-Luc operation is an invasive procedure in which an incision is made in the upper gum above the teeth. A "window" is created to open the sinus so that the tumor can be removed. The procedure is done under a general anesthetic. Because there has been an incision, surgical stitches are made in the mouth, so there is some risk of causing numbness to the upper lip and the adjacent part of the face. This procedure also poses some risk to the health of the gums and teeth at the site of the infection. But if the intent is to remove a tumor, the risk is justified.

External Ethmoidectomy

An open, or external, ethmoidectomy is performed by making an incision on the nose, alongside the eye. The orbital contents (the eye) are then pushed somewhat to one side so as to provide a direct view of the ethmoid sinuses. Like most sinus surgery, the object is to open up the sinus cavity to improve drainage into the nasal airway.

The sphenoid sinus can also be opened through this approach. Fortunately, this operation has essentially been completely replaced by endoscopic intranasal techniques and is only performed rarely today. The risks are the same as those for FESS, but the incidence of complications is higher, and of course the incision will leave a scar.

Open Frontal Sinus Surgery

As with the other sinuses, the need to perform open surgery on the frontal sinuses has dramatically been reduced as a result of the introduction of endoscopic techniques. In recent years, the need for open frontal sinus surgery has been further reduced by the introduction of newer, extended endoscopic techniques and special curved drills. They allow us to open up the frontal sinus using an endoscopic intranasal technique, even when new bone has formed, obstructing the sinus drainage. This technique, called "transseptal frontal sinusotomy," or "endoscopic lothrop procedure," carries a higher risk of CSF leak than standard sinus surgery, but is effective in skilled surgical hands and has further reduced the need for external incisions. It is not, however, an operation typically performed by an average general otolaryngologist.

Despite the fact that the need for open frontal sinus surgery has been dramatically reduced, there are still some situations in which this surgery might be the best approach, particularly if an extended endscopic procedure either fails or is not possible because of unfavorable anatomy. In these cases, one of the operations described below may be recommended:

FRONTAL SINUS OSTEOPLASTY WITH FRONTAL SINUS OBLITERATION. In these two interrelated surgeries, an incision is made either behind the hairline, across the eyebrows, or through the forehead crease, so as to provide access to the frontal sinus in the forehead. After exposing the bone of the frontal sinus, a special power saw is used to cut around the frontal sinus so it can be opened, but the bone over it can be kept in one piece. The sinus can then either be opened widely into the nose from above, or the lining can be removed and the cavity of the sinus filled with fat taken from the abdomen (most of us have more than enough to fill a sinus!). At the end of the operation, the bone is secured back in place and the incisions are closed. Typically, there is significant swelling for a few days, and it is normal to spend a couple of days in the hospital after this type of surgery.

Although this operation sounds pretty brutal, it is not as bad for the patient as it sounds, and is usually quite effective. Additionally, if the incision can be hidden behind the hairline, there are no visible scars. However, even this operation does not guarantee that you will not have further frontal sinus problems; the failure rate for the surgery rises to about 25% over time.

Perhaps one of the biggest disadvantages of this type of surgery is that, if the sinus is obliterated with fat, it is very difficult to image what is happening in the sinus after surgery, with either CT scans or MRIs. Because of this, we do not recommend frontal sinus obliteration when tumors are present in the sinus or when fungus is present. It also means that, if a patient starts to have what seems to be frontal sinus symptoms after an obliteration, it is very difficult to know if inflammation has redeveloped without going back in surgically.

Risks of this type of surgery include the possibility of a visible scar and infection, some numbness in the forehead, and higher risks of CSF leak and double vision than with an endoscopic approach. An osteoplasty with frontal sinus obliteration is indicated when, despite other types of treatment, good drainage is not achieved.

FRONTAL SINUS TREPHINE. In this operation, a small opening is made into the frontal sinus through an incision adjacent to the eyebrow. This opening allows a telescope to be introduced directly into the sinus, for pus to be irrigated out of the sinus, or for a drain to be left in place for a few days. Limited surgery on an outpatient basis can also be performed directly on the sinus through this type of approach.

A frontal sinus trephine is used by some surgeons in conjunction with an endoscopic approach when access is limited through the nose. The scar is usually not visible when it is healed, and the risks of the procedure are few. Occasionally, however, one of the sensation nerves may be damaged by the incision, causing some forehead numbness and, as with other surgery in this region, there is a small risk of double vision or of CSF leak.

Surgeries of the Nose

TURBINATE SURGERY. The turbinates are the baffles of the nose, and vary in size over time as they adjust the airflow through the nose in response to different environmental conditions. The most important, in terms of nasal surgery, are the inferior and middle turbinates. The inferior turbinates change in size most dramatically because of the erectile tissue that they contain, and are therefore most involved in the nasal air-conditioning process. The middle turbinates help to protect the sinuses from pollution and irritants in the air that we breathe.

Because of this continually changing size, one or the other of the inferior turbinates will frequently seem large at one given point in time, such as at the moment that a CT scan or endoscopic examination is performed. However, the bone in the turbinate itself can occasionally become enlarged, such as when the nasal septum is markedly deflected toward the opposite side.

Because the inferior turbinates are a significant factor in controlling airflow, many otolaryngologists will recommend reducing them in size as a way of improving breathing through the nose, and it does frequently help. Indeed, over the years the turbinates have been reduced in size with open surgery, cautery, freezing, laser, and, more recently, with radio frequency (somnoplasty). However, it is important to remember that the turbinates are, in fact, physiological structures that work to ensure the correct airflow through the nose and help to create a large surface area for the warming, humidification, and purification of the air. For this reason, I do not advocate performing inferior turbinate surgery unless it is absolutely essential—for instance, when the bone of one turbinate has enlarged to the point that the septum cannot be replaced to the midline of the nose. Even then, I believe any turbinate surgery should be performed conservatively. Because of the current level of accuracy in testing, we find few demonstrable harmful effects even from complete inferior turbinate removal. Still, occasionally, one of the complaints of too much turbinate removal is nasal obstruction, because increasing the size of the nasal cavity can actually increase resistance if it causes turbulent airflow through the nose. When all the turbinates are surgically removed, the nose becomes a wide cavity, but it is susceptible to the formation of crusts and frequently feels obstructed. There is also a significantly increased risk of sinusitis, and mucus clearance by the cilia will be unlikely to ever return to normal. This condition has been referred to as the "Empty Nose Syndrome," and is very uncomfortable for the patient. There is no effective way of correcting it surgically and rebuilding the turbinates if they have been removed surgically.

The middle turbinates lie close to the ethmoid sinuses and, in the past, were sometimes routinely removed during an ethmoidectomy. However, because they also participate in directing airflow and protecting the sinuses, they are probably best left intact during surgery unless they are significantly diseased (have nasal polyps, for instance) or very inflamed.

SEPTOPLASTY. Septoplasty is a surgical procedure used to correct a deviated septum. As we discussed in Chapter 8, very few people have a perfectly formed septum but, in some people, the septum has enough of an abnormality that it interferes with breathing. This abnormality may be congenital (something you're born with), or the result of an injury such as a broken nose.

Septal surgery can usually be performed on an outpatient basis and either a general or a local anesthetic may be used. It can also be combined with FESS when necessary. The incision is made inside the nose, and the correction of the septal deformities may either be done under external vision with a headlight or, increasingly, under endoscopic visualization. In these procedures, the septum may be repaired and replaced, or portions of it may be removed entirely. Sometimes a septoplasty is combined with a rhinoplasty, in which the shape of the nose is altered. As with sinus surgery, it is less common today to perform tight nasal packing following a septoplasty than it was 20 years ago. Frequently, only small sponges are placed, and they are removed in one to two days.

The nasal cartilage has some memory and, when it is straightened, it might tend to bend back to its original position. Accordingly, the septum is rarely 100 percent straight, even following surgery. The septum also helps to provide support to the tip of the nose. The key to the success of this surgery is for the surgeon to straighten the septum sufficiently without, at the same time, causing any loss of support to the tip of the nose.

Most people who have had a septoplasty will have a little swelling around the eyes, a small amount of bleeding, headache, and some puffiness. However, complications from septoplasty are uncommon. Decreased sense of smell, alteration in the shape of the nose, or some numbness in the front teeth are uncommon complications. Occasionally, septal surgery can also cause a hole to develop through the nasal septum (septal perforation). Many septal perforations are asymptomatic but, occasionally, they can cause crusting, bleeding, or even a feeling of nasal obstruction. Septal perforations can be repaired with grafts from other parts of the body.

RHINOPLASTY. Rhinoplasty (sometimes called aesthetic nasal surgery) is surgery to the nose either to correct a malformation in the nose, or as a form of plastic surgery intended to change the shape of the nose for cosmetic purposes. If the object is to reshape the nose, the surgeon lifts the skin of the patient and removes or rearranges the bone and cartilage. The skin is then re-draped over the newly created frame. For this procedure, the patient is often given a general anesthetic. The recovery period and the risks are somewhat greater for rhinoplasty than for septoplasty (see above); the swelling is usually significantly more severe, there may be some bruising, and there is always the risk that the cosmetic result may not be the one desired.

Surgeries of the Throat

ADENOIDECTOMY. As we discussed in Chapter 2, the adenoids are glands located in the nasopharynx and are composed primarily of lymph tissue. While the adenoids play an important role in fighting infections in infants and young children, as the immune system becomes more mature, the adenoids generally shrink and typically disappear by the time a person reaches adulthood. Sometimes, however, for reasons we don't completely understand, they don't shrink and may become inflamed and infected, causing pain and discomfort. Even in children, they sometimes contribute to the development of fluid in the ear, or cause nasal obstruction, snoring, and even sleep disturbance. In these cases, an adenoidectomy may be recommended.

Sometimes performed in conjunction with a tonsillectomy, this procedure is usually done under general anesthetic. A small instrument is inserted into the mouth to prop it open. Then, the adenoids are removed either with a curette or a microdebrider. Another technique is to cauterize the adenoids instead of removing them. Unless complications occur, this procedure is performed in less than an hour and the patient can go home in a few hours. Other than the possibility of a sore throat for several days, there are usually very few complications following this surgery. Risks of the surgery include bleeding and, rarely, the risk of causing some change in the child's voice (hypernasality), at least until the patient has learned to adapt, creating additional movement of the palate to compensate for the additional space.

TONSILLECTOMY. The tonsils are clumps of tissues located on either side of the throat next to the soft palate. Like the adenoids, the tonsils are thought to exist primarily to help infants and small children fight infection. In most people, the tonsils cause little trouble, but in other children and adults they may, like the adenoids, become inflamed and painful and result in recurrent tonsillitis. If pain and inflammation are recurrent, a doctor may recommend a tonsillectomy. The procedure is very similar to an adenoidectomy. However, the recovery period is significantly longer. There is typically a severe sore throat, and swallowing may be quite painful for one to two weeks.

Does Sinus Surgery Always Work?

The purpose of surgery is to clear the airways and to correct any congenital malformations or growths in the nose or sinus cavities. Because rhinosinusitis is generally caused by an inflammation in the mucus membranes, and the mucus membranes at the periphery of the sinuses are still there after surgery, the infection can come back. So, in that sense, surgery seldom *cures* rhinosinusitis. Its purpose, instead, is to help eliminate the problems that have made the infections more likely to occur.

Therefore, for surgery to be effective, the patient must continue to be conscientious about caring for the nose and sinus cavities.

Here are some steps you should take to help assure that your rhinosinusitis doesn't recur:

1. Manage your allergies.
2. Avoid smoking and secondhand smoke.

3. Continue to use your medications as directed, and irrigate your nose as instructed by your physician.
4. Keep your house free from dust and molds
5. Alert your doctor at the first sign of infection
6. Follow your sense of smell. A decrease in your sense of smell can be an early sign of inflammation returning to the sinus area.

WHAT IF SURGERY DOESN'T WORK? Although sinus surgery, particularly endoscopic surgery, has a very high rate of success, as with all medical treatments there are always cases in which the procedure does not produce the desired effect. If surgery has not decreased the incidence of chronic rhinosinusitis, the doctor will usually then consider one of the following options:

1. A different course of antibiotic therapy, trying a new antibiotic or another antibiotic technique, such as administering it intravenously. In some cases, an antifungal medication may be recommended, either administered orally or as irrigation.
2. Another type of surgery
3. A different type of irrigation, or topically applied medications
4. A course of oral steroids
5. Consultation with a subspecialty-trained nasal and sinus specialist (rhinologist)

15

COMPLEMENTARY AND ALTERNATIVE MEDICINE AND THERAPIES
Nontraditional Choices

OR MANY YEARS "ALTERNATIVE" MEDICINE was anything mainstream doctors didn't understand or approve of. Today, many doctors are still skeptical, but are beginning to view some forms of alternative medicine as another valid choice. Within the last 10 years or so, some mainstream doctors, hospitals, and clinics have even begun to include therapies such as acupuncture, therapeutic massage, and various kinds of relaxation techniques within their range of services, because there is increasing recognition that an individual's overall state of health and well-being may play a significant role in many diseases.

The Origins of Alternative Medicine

For as long as there has been life on Earth, there has been illness and injury. And for as long as there have been human illnesses and injuries, people have searched for ways to cure and treat them. For our earliest ancestors, we can only assume that finding treatments that worked was pretty much a matter of trial and error. The remedies that didn't work were probably buried along with the unfortunate patient. The remedies that did work were passed along to future generations. Those who had the best record at providing cures and treatments on a more permanent basis formed the foundation of the science of medicine. People who practiced the healing arts also soon began to mix the herbs and other substances that had proven effective in prior generations to achieve an even better outcome. They became, in effect, the world's first pharmacists.

Prescientific Theories of Medicine

Since healing was often considered a miracle—and sometimes magic—many cultures considered healers and healing to have a spiritual and religious component. Therefore, early on, the practice of medicine took on a spiritual point of view as potions, powders, and even prayers were thought to be effective in healing ailments.

Early philosophical works based on the understanding of the human body also led to a belief that the body contained some sort of inner energy. All bodily functions were assumed to be affected positively or negatively by the natural elements that people could experience firsthand, such as air, water, earth, and fire.

The Greek philosopher Hippocrates believed that the body was made up of four "humors"—blood, phlegm, yellow bile, and black bile—and that an imbalance of these humors was the basis for disease. Others at that time, however, thought that disease was sent by the gods, and thus all cures could only be determined by them.

When the Romans conquered the Greeks, they adopted these ideas. The Romans also began to experiment with herbs and other remedies, and even came to understand that cleanliness led to healthier lives. Out of this belief system came the notion of "civilized society," which included the creation of baths, aqueducts and sophisticated sewer systems.

To these basic beliefs were added further philosophical interpretations of what forces were responsible for life and bodily functions. Galen, a philosopher and physician born in 129 AD, became the unchallenged authority on medicine for the next thousand years. Although not religious himself, he nonetheless regarded the body as the instrument of the soul and believed that "pneuma" (breath and air) formed the fundamental principal of life.

Origins of Mainstream Medicine

In the sixteenth century, English physician William Harvey discovered that circulation of blood through the body was actually the basic "humor", or life-sustaining function. Before long, these ideas developed into a formal belief system that, along with pharmacoepia (the known inventory of drugs, chemicals, and treatments), shaped the mainstream practice of medicine.

A huge medical advance, vaccination against disease, was made in 1798 by Edward Jenner, who developed a vaccine for smallpox. By the 1930s, there were vaccines for rabies, plague, diptheria, pertussis, tuberculosis, tetanus, and yellow fever; in the 1950s and 1960s, vaccines were developed for polio, measles, and mumps; and finally, in the 1970s and early 1980s, there were vaccines for rubella and hepatitis B. In 1928, Scottish scientist Alexander Fleming discovered penicillin; prior to that, diseases caused by bacteria and viruses, like measles, mumps, diphtheria, and smallpox killed thousands of people each year. So, when scientists began to formulate vaccines and increasingly effective medicines for other ailments, it is little wonder people began to abandon folk cures in favor of the "miracle cures" that appeared (and keep appearing) on the market. Other medical breakthroughs included Louis Pasteur's discovery in the mid-1800s that germs cause disease, and the discovery of insulin in 1922 by Frederick Banting and Charles Best.

All of these discoveries, combined with the widespread availability of clean water, made a tremendous impact on public health. No wonder traditional healers and medicines were considered by many as hopelessly old-fashioned and ineffective. For most Americans, the best medicine was created by a pharmaceutical company, and the best place for treatment was in a nice clean hospital.

In developed countries, formally trained physicians represent the mainstream practice of medicine today. They are educated in medical schools and then serve an apprenticeship in which they study with those who have more experience. In mainstream medicine, physicians rely on treatments and medicines that have stood the test of time and have been formally approved for use in our country, by agencies like the FDA and are recommended by organizations within the various medical specialties.

A Renewed Interest in Herbal Medicines

In the 1960s, however, there was a backlash of sorts. Young adults began to rebel against what they considered the overly materialistic lifestyles of their parents and, along with their back-to-a-simpler-life philosophy, came a renewed interest in all things natural, including foods and medicines. While, as they aged, most 1960s hippies became disillusioned with the harsh realities of subsistence farming and communal lifestyle, many brought with them into middle age the belief that "natural" foods and medicines are somehow superior to those produced "chemically."

Over time, we have begun to learn that alternatives to mainstream medicine, although not a replacement, can be helpful as an adjunctive approach to treating some bodily ailments. In many medical practices and hospitals, these alternative treatments are now known as "complementary," since they are used in addition to drugs, surgery, and other more mainstream therapies. However, in many cultures, particularly in developing nations, what we still consider largely "alternative" is what constitutes the majority of medical practice.

According to a recent study conducted by the Indiana University School of Medicine, every year nearly 60 million Americans are using alternative therapies at a cost of $13.7 billion, and the number of annual visits to providers of alternative medicine may actually exceed the number of visits to primary care physicians. For many years there was very little interest in studying the effect of alternative therapies. However, the increased interest in these medicines by consumers has now resulted in greater attention to how various alternative therapies may interact with other mainstream drugs and treatments. It is also increasingly important that physicians be aware of the different types of alternative treatments, the scientific evidence surrounding those treatments, and their potential interactions with other medical therapies they may be prescribing. Most medical and nursing/health care providers/schools are now training physicians to understand other philosophical bases for the treatment of disease. Furthermore, a large number of studies are emerging that specifically look at the effect alternative medicines have on patient well-being in both physical and mental health.

Why Turn to Alternative Medicine?

A primary complaint of many patients is that traditional medicine treats only the problem, not the patient—that is, the emphasis is upon diagnosing and curing your disease or disorder, but not on preventing it or dealing with the effects it may have on other areas of your life. Scientifically-based medicine has naturally been biased toward that which is easily measured accurately and scientifically, and has turned away from more complex factors and interactions such as the overall feeling of well-being, the influence of stress, depression, and mental health. Especially for chronic conditions in which many different factors come into play and for which mainstream medicine offers no cure, such as allergies, asthma, and sinusitis, the holistic approach of alternative medicine can be helpful.

Another factor in the increased awareness of alternative medicine is that the United States is a nation of immigrants. Because of this, many patients come from cultures where medical treatment is based on very different philosophies and where medicine is practiced quite differently. This influx of cultural differences also inadvertently contributes to the way ailments are treated in the United States. For example, Chinese immigrants have brought with them a whole new collection of Asian medicines that, until recently, have been poorly understood in our culture.

Additionally, there will always be people that are skeptical of the "chemical" medicines that physicians typically prescribe. Some people are afraid of medicines, regardless of the source. Other patients are particularly skeptical if the treatment is pharmacologically produced. To meet the demand for what they consider more "natural" treatments, some people (and an increasing number of large companies) have concocted medications from plants and a variety of other substances. This unfortunately, has become a problem in the United States and other countries because some manufacturers of these alternative medicines are now marketing products that have not been scientifically proven to help and that can actually harm you. In other words, "natural" does not necessarily mean "good for you."

For one or more of these reasons, many people often seek treatment from alternative medicines and practitioners of alternative therapies. Additionally, physicians may be more inclined to recommend alternative therapies, as new evidence continues to come to light about the important interplay between overall bodily and mental health and the effects on the immune system and specific diseases.

It is likely that physicians and scientists will continue to study such alternative therapies in large patient populations to prove (or disprove) their efficacy. It also seems probable that more and more beneficial alternative therapies will someday be incorporated into mainstream medicine.

What Are Some of These Alternative Medicines and Therapies?

Every culture has developed a slightly different approach to treating injury and illness. Although there are many varieties of alternative medicines including Reiki, Ayurveda, reflexology, and so on, among the most popular are Chinese medicine, homeopathy, naturopathy, aromatherapy, and herbal medicines.

CHINESE MEDICINE. Chinese medicine, which has been practiced for at least 5,000 years, is based on the belief that in all of nature there are opposing forces—night and day, hot and cold, up and down, and so on. These opposing forces are known as the yin and yang. Most of us are familiar with the symbol that is commonly used to illustrate this concept.

The yin is the "dark" side of nature, the yang the "light." As with every other living thing, the human body is considered to have both yin and yang qualities. The liver, for example, is dark and solid and is considered a yin organ, while the sinuses, since they are hollow, are considered to be yang. Although it takes many years of study to fully understand the intricacies of Chinese medicine, in general, it can be said that the goal of treatment is to help the patient achieve a balance between the yin and yang.

Another important element of Chinese medicine is that it is holistic. Those who practice Chinese medicine believe that it is impossible to separate the physical from the spiritual, emotional, and mental aspects of the individual. Thus, all treatment is directed at the whole person, not just a particular disease or complaint.

Like those who practice Western medicine, practitioners of Chinese medicine generally perform a physical examination, but do so in quite a different way from Western doctors, relying heavily upon taking the pulse in different areas, studying the tongue, and touching the body to determine temperature and moisture.

If you seek help for your sinusitis from a Chinese doctor, a Chinese medicine will probably be prescribed. These medicines may come in the form of a combination of herbs and plants that you will take as tablets or liquid or make into a tea. For most American tastes, Chinese medicinal teas take some getting used to. A Chinese doctor may also recommend that you try acupuncture.

ACUPUNCTURE. Acupuncture is based on the belief that every living thing contains a life force known as ch'i (pronounced *chee*). Ch'i flows along 14 invisible, interconnected "meridians" that exist on each side of the body and crisscross the arms, legs, trunk, and head, and flow through the muscles.

There are 360 points along these meridians. Where the meridians come to the surface of the skin, acupuncture points are created. Because each meridian is connected to one or more organs, stimulating one or more of the acupuncture points can positively impact that organ. Since energy is constantly flowing along the meridians, an interruption or imbalance in the flow of ch'i upsets the balance of the yin and yang and can cause discomfort or illness. Application of acupuncture restores the balance. In China, the belief in the effectiveness of acupuncture is so widespread that is even used as an anesthetic for patients undergoing major surgery.

Although no one knows for sure exactly how acupuncture works, one theory is that application of acupuncture needles causes a release of endorphins in the brain. Endorphins are naturally produced polypeptide (protein) brain substances that can have the same effect as chemical narcotics by binding to opiate receptors, thereby alleviating pain. There is also some evidence that stimulating acupoints dissipates lactic acid in the muscles. (In Chinese medicine, the accumulation of carbon monoxide and lactic acid in the muscles is thought to be caused by an imbalance in the influence of the five elements: wood, fire, earth, water, and metal.) Another theory is that acupuncture raises the levels of triglycerides, hormones, prostaglandins, white blood cells, and gamma globulin. Yet another theory is that acupuncture causes a release of such vasodilators as histamines, which dilate the blood vessels.

Whatever the actual mechanism, acupuncture is now more widely accepted than ever before as an effective alternative or complementary therapy. Because acupuncture needles are very thin, acupuncture is a relatively painless procedure.

There are specific acupuncture treatments for rhinosinusitis. However, their efficacy has not studied scientifically and their value therefore remains uncertain.

ACUPRESSURE. Acupressure is based on the same principles as acupuncture. The difference is that instead of inserting needles into the acupuncture points, pressure is applied to that point for a specific period of time. One of the advantages of acupressure is that a patient can be trained to do this therapy for him- or herself. As in acupuncture, the pressure points that affect various organs are along the meridians that exist throughout the body.

HOMEOPATHY. Homeopathy (from "homeo" meaning similar and "pathos" meaning disease in Latin and Greek) was founded by a German, Samuel Christian Hahnemann, in the late 1700s. Hahnemann's philosophy was that symptoms of a disease were signs of the body's attempt to resist disease; he called this suppression. He believed the medical practitioners of his time were primarily concerned with addressing symptoms of diseases rather than the root cause of the symptoms, and that the human body was usually capable of curing itself if given the right stimulation in the form of what he called bioenergetic medicines. These medicines were minute amounts of plant, animal, and mineral substances that would, in higher dosages, be toxic or cause the symptoms of a disease.

Homeopathy, as it applies to sinusitis, theorizes that conventional medicines, such as antibiotics, weaken the immune system and lead to an overgrowth of candida, a yeast that can both directly and indirectly worsen sinusitis. By contrast, once the immune system is correctly stimulated by homeopathic medicines, it will return the body to homeostasis—the same sort of balanced state that Chinese medicine tries to achieve. Hahnemann tested his remedies on healthy people to produce symptoms, figuring that the same remedy, in a smaller dosage, would cure those same symptoms in a person who was ill.

Since homeopathy takes a holistic approach to medicine, the homeopathic healer views the patient as a whole person, taking into account everything that is going on in that person's life. Thus, homeopathic remedies, like Chinese herbs, are prescribed on an individual basis.

Homeopathic remedies come in many forms—tablets, pellets, granules, powders, liquids, ointments, oils, gels, sprays, and soaps. Since these remedies contain only minute quantities of basic ingredients, potency is measured by the amount of dilution. Homeopathic medicines are unlike Western medicines in that, the more diluted they are, the more potent they are thought to be.

Homeopathic medicines are considered to be especially effective for people with chronic diseases like rhinosinusitis. Many of these preparations are sold in health food stores. No conclusive scientific data has supported their use. However, because the active herb is so diluted, the relative risk to the consumer is probably low.

NATUROPATHY. As its name suggests, naturopathy is based on the theory that our bodies can best heal themselves; that is, regain the inner balance that restores health through "natural" activities like a diet of unprocessed foods, exercise, a clean environment, and hydrotherapy. Naturopathic healers, unlike homeopathic healers, take advantage of Western diagnostic methods such as imaging and testing. Although some minor surgeries are considered acceptable, naturopaths do not believe in major surgery or the use of most synthetic drugs. They do recognize the value of other holistic therapies and remedies such as acupuncture, Chinese medicine, and homeopathy.

In treating sinusitis, naturopaths recommend the same types of lifestyle changes as most Western physicians, including eating small meals that are low in fat. They also recommend cessation of smoking and avoidance of carbonated drinks.

The Evolution from Natural to Chemical to Synthetic

Since the debate about avoiding "chemical" products is confusing to many people, it deserves some discussion.

So what, really, is the difference between natural and chemical medicines?

First, it should be noted that most medicines that we use today either have been developed using natural products. The heart drug digitalis is derived from foxglove; lotions made with aloe vera soothe the pain of sunburn; the bark of the yew tree is the source of the cancer drug, Taxol.

From the beginning, however, few healers prescribed these natural remedies in their natural state. The first change to most natural remedies was aesthetic. Even the earliest healers realized that a medicine wasn't much good if the patient wouldn't take it. So, since many herbal cures were somewhat less than palatable, these healers began to mix these natural substances with alcohol, spices, and perfumes and to dye them more attractive colors.

As time went on, those formulating medicines also began to address other issues.

PURITY. The first of these issues was purity. Even though, until the mid-1800s, doctors didn't have the faintest idea about what caused infection, they did seem to understand that using "natural" things meant that they were getting a lot of cross-contamination. It was difficult to grind up a plant to get the desired medicinal effect without also ending up with other effects, sometimes harmful, produced by other parts of the plant. As they began to understand the chemistry of the substances they were using, scientists began to be able to isolate just what the desired ingredient was. Beginning (in most cases) in the 1800s, after scientists isolated an ingredient, they than figured out how to produce these medicines "synthetically", thus being able to reliably separate out from the natural source just those ingredients they needed.

DOSAGE. In its natural state, the medicinal level of many herbs and other plants is highly unpredictable, making correct dosage an important issue. Different strains of a plant or plants grown in different soils may produce a wide variety of different potencies. And, without chemical testing, there was no way to be sure except by trial and error. As soon as a drug could be produced synthetically, each dose could be assured to be identical.

AVAILABILITY, CONVENIENCE, AND COST. Medicines were one of the first products to be traded internationally, as explorers brought back with them the "magic potions" they had found on their travels. While such drugs were often effective, they were not only expensive to import, but were often difficult to obtain. The ability to produce them synthetically assured a consistent, available, cost-effective supply.

DIRECT ACTION AND SIDE EFFECTS. Most botanicals contain not just one, but many compounds, which may have a variety of effects and, while curing one problem, another was sometimes created. For example, a certain medicinal tea might work well to fight a fever, but might also be a powerful laxative. Using the herb in its natural state, it was impossible to separate the two effects. Isolating the different elements of the drugs contained in the tea, and finding out each of their different properties and effects, allowed a drug to be administered to work directly on one problem without causing another.

Also, herbs in their natural state could cause unpleasant side effects when the recipient was allergic to one of the many active ingredients in the remedy. By isolating the desired active ingredient, synthetic drugs can be formulated to eliminate side effects.

REGULATION. Throughout most of history, the production of medicines was largely unregulated. The best a patient could hope for was a reputable and competent pharmacist or doctor. If neither of them was reputable or competent, there was little recourse. Because there were no central testing facilities, anyone could mix up just about anything and, providing it didn't kill anyone, get by with selling it to the unsuspecting public.

For example, traveling "medicine shows" were big attractions during the 1800s in this country. Although the medicines sold by these itinerant entertainers were usually mostly alcohol, or in some cases cocaine or morphine, "the medicine man" had left town days before the patient realized that that happy feeling obtained from the drug wasn't doing much to solve the initial problem. Additionally, there was virtually no inspection of drugs, so even efficacious drugs were often contaminated.

The US government began to regulate drugs as early as 1862, with the hiring of a single chemist in the US Department of Agriculture. Prior to this time, the regulation of drugs, such as it was, rested with the states. In 1906, the Federal Food and Drugs Act created the modern FDA.

Now this giant bureaucracy includes more than 9,000 employees and has an annual budget of more than $1 billion. In addition to approving drugs, the agency also regulates medical devices, food and color additives, infant formulas, and animal drugs, and monitors the manufacture, import, transport, storage, and sale of $1 trillion worth of products. Today, all prescription drugs sold by US manufacturers must be approved by the FDA before they may be sold to the public.

Aromatherapy

Because our sense of smell is such an important part of our lives, particular aromas have a strong emotional impact on most people. Although all organic matter has an aroma, some of which are much stronger than others, the aromas used in aromatherapy are generally produced from pure essential oils. These are highly-concentrated extracts that are heated, burned as candles, or added to hot bath water. As discussed in Chapter 10, breathing in warm, moist air and oils such as menthol and eucalyptus is often a highly effective way to relieve sinus congestion.

Herbal Medicines and Food Supplements

Although the Chinese were early advocates of herbal medicines, they may not have been the first nor certainly, are they the only culture to use them. In fact, in the Middle East, India, Egypt, Greece, and Rome, the use of herbal medicines has always been the primary system of treatment. American Indians also have a strong healing tradition that includes both the spiritual and religious elements of Asian medicine ,as well as a pharmacoepia of herbal medicines. It is estimated that up to 80 percent of the world's population still depends primarily on herbal remedies. In the past as well as now, the most common method of delivering these medicines is in the form of a tea or a soup, although they were (and are) still given as infusions, decoctions, compresses, or poultices. An infusion is made by pouring boiling water over the herbs; a decoction is made by simmering herbs (or other substances like roots or bark) in water. Compresses are applied by soaking a cloth in the liquid produced by an infusion or decoction. A poultice is created by applying a fresh herb directly to an area of the body and covering it with a bandage or cloth.

In Chinese medicine, unlike many Western remedies, the combinations of herbs can be formulated to cure several things at once.

Most Chinese herbs are made into strong teas and, as mentioned earlier, the taste takes some getting used to by most people who have not grown up with it.

Herbal Remedies

Herbal remedies were among the first medicines in history and are still used extensively in many cultures, including our own. Some herbalists believe that treatment for sinusitis should be both indirect and direct. For example, some believe that overproduction of mucus is an attempt by the body to discharge waste material that is not properly eliminated through digestion or through the skin. An "indirect" treatment for this would be to prescribe a laxative or diuretic. Another idea is that an emotional state can sometimes bring on an attack of sinusitis and that crying, for example, can free "blocked energy" and thus help the sinuses to drain.

Herbal remedies suggested in the treatment of rhinosinusitis include anise, bitter orange oil, cat's claw, dandelion, echinacea, garlic, ginko biloba, horseradish, goldenseal root, lavender, and vitamins A, B complex and C, and minerals such as zinc.

Again, it is important that, if you take any herbal medications, you discuss these with your physician because of the potential interactions that they may have with prescribed medications. Some herbs, for instance, thin the blood and can therefore cause excessive bleeding during surgery.

Dietary Remedies

In addition to herbs, healers in most societies have traditionally recommended that specific foods either be eaten or avoided in order to treat a particular disorder. While in general most physicians now advocate a well-balanced diet combined with exercise, other practitioners of "natural healing" suggest some of the following tips for treating sinusitis. If a patient has a fever, it is suggested that all solid foods be avoided in favor of a diluted version of fresh fruit and vegetable juices (50 percent juice to 50 percent water). Carrot, cucumber, beet, and spinach juice are particularly recommended. As the fever subsides, the patient should then adopt a low-calorie raw fruit-and-vegetable diet along with raw fruit juice. After the symptoms subside, the patient can then add seeds, nuts, grains, vegetables, and fruit. We recommend that anyone suffering from sinusitis avoid fried and starchy foods, white sugar, white flour, rice, macaroni products, sweets, meat, and strong spices. It is popularly believed that milk and milk products increase mucus production and, therefore, are best avoided in patients with sinus problems. However, one study that looked at this issue did not find any evidence to support an increase in mucus production or change in mucus consistency brought on by dairy products. Indeed, some dietary healers have recommended that patients should drink a lot of milk to overcome inflammation of the sinuses, but should avoid citrus fruits.

Other practitioners of dietary remedies suggest a fruit fast for several days, hot lemon drinks, mustard, and aromatic herbs.

Food Supplements

Although acute bacterial sinusitis is probably best treated with antibiotics, advocates of "natural remedies" often recommend the use of various nutritional supplements, both to reduce the tendency toward infection and to increase the immune response. These products include bee pollen, bormelian, garlic, oibas oil, menthol, and zinc.

Almost every natural food store and many pharmacies and groceries now contain a wide variety of food supplements whose manufacturers make many claims about their benefits. Thus, the consumer is often presented with a dizzying array of all kinds of products, with conflicting claims about what supplement does what. As we have stressed throughout this book, if you are contemplating taking *anything* for your rhinosinusitis—including over-the-counter medications, herbs, vitamins or supplements, you should consult your doctor before you do. Remember, just because something is natural doesn't mean it won't react with other medications you are taking.

More than 20,000 vitamins, herbs, and minerals now on the market are not subject to FDA monitoring. Manufacturers of these products are not required to provide either information about the contents of these compounds or the method of preparation. Unlike other drugs, they do not require the mention of possible side effects or any proof of efficacy. Some, like those offered in the old-time medicine shows, provide results by the addition of caffeine or alcohol. Most have not been scientifically tested.

In addition, many of these products are imported so there is no way of knowing how they were grown, harvested, or stored or what pesticides may have been used on them.

Also, remember that "natural" doesn't necessarily mean safe. Some herbs that grow naturally, perhaps even in your own backyard, are very dangerous. Other herbs may be safe, but completely useless in treating disease or discomfort.

Buying Drugs from the Internet

These days, it is almost impossible to collect your e-mail from the Internet without being barraged with advertisements for drugs and other types of therapies. Some online merchants offer alternative types of medications such as various kinds of food supplements. Others offer brand-name medicines. While the prices of these medications may seem very attractive, remember that there is no way to tell for sure where these drugs originated or whether or not they are counterfeit, even if the packages bear brand names. Some online suppliers are legitimate, but many are not. Before buying drugs or other remedies from the Internet, consult your doctor to make sure you will be getting what you pay for.

Consult Your Doctor Before Using an Alternative Drug or Therapy

Otolaryngologists and other medical professionals understand that the treatment of disease is a very individual thing. Patients with the same symptoms often respond very differently to the medications and lifestyle changes that are recommended by doctors. Some patients may well benefit from some of the complementary or alternative medications or therapies that have been discussed in this chapter. Because all medications and therapies have the potential to interact with one another, however, before trying any of these alternative or complementary regimens, you should certainly discuss this idea with your doctor. If you are using any of these products or therapies now, you should certainly tell your doctor about them as you are discussing what the most appropriate treatment will be for your rhinosinusitis.

16

PREVENTION

What You Can Do to Avoid Symptoms

O BVIOUSLY, THE BEST "CURE" FOR ANY disease is to avoid getting it in the first place. But because rhinosinusitis is acquired primarily by one of life's major necessities—breathing—it is not always easy to prevent. Fortunately, however, there are some precautions you can take to avoid having many common elements in the environment negatively affect your sinuses.

Pollution

Air pollution, one of the unfortunate side effects of living in an industrial society, is undisputedly one of the major causes of rhinosinusitis. In fact, studies suggest that pollution is even more of a factor in rhinosinusitis than allergies. When it comes to air pollution, the good news is that the nose is an excellent air conditioner and air purifier, so only a very small amount of the pollutants that we breathe in ever reach the lower airways and the lungs. The bad news is that the brunt of these pollutants and particles are absorbed by the nose, making it susceptible to inflammation and infection and, over time, causing the potential for permanent changes in the lining mucosa.

While there may not be much that you can do about outdoor air pollution (other than getting rid of that gas-guzzler SUV!), there are things that you can do about indoor air pollution. Included are not allowing anyone to smoke indoors, avoiding open fires and unvented gas fireplaces, avoiding exposure to chemicals, paint, new carpets, and airborne dust.

Viruses, Bacteria, Fungi, and Molds

As we discussed in Chapter 7, viruses, bacteria, fungi, and molds are the most common infectious causes of rhinosinusitis. Since all of these exist in virtually every climate on Earth, it is impossible to avoid all contact with them. (In the case of bacteria, you would certainly not want to anyway, since bacteria are, on the whole, primarily beneficial to humans.) However, there are certain precautions you should take regarding them to reduce the symptoms of rhinosinusitis.

VIRUSES. Viral infections frequently precede bacterial infections, and are a major factor in predisposing an individual toward them. While viral upper respiratory infections are more common in winter, they can occur any time of the year in any climate and can cause varying degrees of symptoms, from passing essentially unnoticed to being very debilitating for several days.

Viruses are also more likely to cause infections in people who are under stress. In fact, studies have shown that when volunteers are directly inoculated with the cold virus, and everyone in the study can be shown to have been infected, the chances of having symptoms are significantly greater among those experiencing stress. Thus it follows that, if you can reduce the stress in your life, you can significantly reduce the risk of contracting rhinosinusitis from viruses.

Additionally, since bacterial infections typically follow viral infections, dealing with the lifestyle issues discussed in this chapter should also have an effect on the incidence of bacterial sinusitis.

Viruses can be passed from one person to another through coughing or sneezing; however, getting viruses on your hands and then transferring the viruses to the eyes, nose or mouth are probably more likely to spread them. Regular hand washing is therefore very important in preventing upper respiratory infections, particularly if you are handling items that have been handled by someone who has a cold, or who is incubating a cold. Unfortunately, no matter how careful you are when you are around other people, viral infections cannot be completely avoided.

BACTERIA. Most bacterial infections either follow a viral infection or are a result of some other factor (such as pollution) that interferes with the ability of mucous membranes to clear mucus. Many people try to protect the nose from bacteria, but in actuality this is not the most important factor in reducing the incidence of bacterial infections.

While bacteria can grow just about anyplace where there are nutrients and water, they seem to be particularly fond of warm, moist places such as inflamed nasal passages with poor mucociliary clearance.

Bacteria also reproduce quickly. In the home, the kitchen, bathroom, and basement are probably the areas that host the most disease-causing (pathogenic) bacteria. If you are susceptible to bacterial rhinosinusitis, you should make an extra effort to keep these areas of you home clean and dry (more about this later in this chapter).

Bacteria, like viruses, also spread quickly from person to person, primarily through hand contact. One of the easiest ways to avoid bacterial infection is to wash your hands frequently, particularly after using the bathroom, touching other people, or touching items frequented by other people, such as handrails, phones, or merchandise in a store. Because it is not always easy to find soap and water, it is a good idea to carry with you one of the many "waterless" antibacterial hand cleaners now on the market.

It is particularly important for rhinosinusitis sufferers to remember that bacteria can be spread by the use of nasal sprays and irrigations. Although most tap water typically does not have significant bacteria in it, we still recommend the use of sterile (boiled) water for nasal irrigations since occasional, and sometimes difficult to treat, infections have occurred from using tap water.

Additionally, nasal sprays should not be shared with other people. Even when they are not shared, it is probably a good idea to run the tip under hot water after each use. If you use a nasal irrigation, the solution should only be kept a few days once a sterile container has been opened, and any devices used to irrigate the nose should be sterilized and routinely replaced.

FUNGI AND MOLDS. Fungi, like bacteria, are present all around us, and are a vital part of our ecosystem. Fungi break down dead organic material, providing nutrients for other plants, and disposing of nature's waste products. Fungi consist of foods like mushrooms and, since yeast is also a type of fungi, allow us to bake bread and make beer and champagne. The downside, for humans, is that fungi also cause ringworm, athlete's foot, and some forms of rhinosinusitis. Also, like bacteria, fungi like to grow in warm, moist places.

Molds are among the estimated 100,000 types of fungi. Molds reproduce asexually by sending spores into the atmosphere. Thus, molds frequently exist in places where air is constantly moving, such as the air ducts in buildings. Unlike most bacteria, molds can remain dormant for extended periods and then become active if they are exposed to water.

Although most of us are familiar with the kinds of molds that are easily seen, like those that grow on stale bread or in a shower stall, many molds are microscopic, and therefore impossible for us to see with the naked eye. Those mold species that seem to cause the most problems for rhinosinusitis sufferers are *Altenaria, Aspergillus, Penicillium, Stachybotrys, Chartarum,* and *Trichoderma.* The role that yeast (candida) may play in chronic rhinosinusitis is, at this stage, not known.

The one thing most molds have in common is that they prefer damp places, so if you are sensitive to molds or have chronic sinusitis, you must make a special effort to keep your home as clean and dry as possible. If you see a small amount of mold on a wall, it is likely that there is a significantly greater amount in the same place that you do not see.

KITCHENS. Molds commonly grow in kitchens, and one of the places molds are most frequently found is in the cabinet under the sink or in the evaporation pan under frost-free refrigerators. Molds especially like to grow in garbage containers where food scraps are present. For these reasons, it is not a good idea to keep your kitchen trash container in the cabinet under the sink.

You should also pay special attention to cutting boards and kitchen cabinets and always use a clean sponge or cloth to wipe surfaces where food has been prepared. The word "clean" is key here, since one of the best ways to spread molds and bacteria in the kitchen is by wiping your hands, cooking utensils, silverware, and cabinets with sponges or cloths that are contaminated with them.

Because cooking releases moisture into the atmosphere, it is also a good idea to install an exhaust fan in the kitchen and always use it when cooking, particularly when boiling food in an open container.

BATHROOMS. In bathrooms, mold not only accumulates in the places where you can see it, like the shower stall, but also frequently in bathroom carpeting. If you are sensitive to molds, it is probably a good idea not to have carpeting in your bathroom. If you use area rugs or bath mats in your bathroom, be sure to wash them frequently. Molds also like to grow on shower curtains, so they should also be washed often.

BASEMENTS. Molds are also frequently found in basements that tend to accumulate moisture, so basement carpets often are full of molds. Even though the carpet itself may seem dry and free of mold, mold often grows in the carpet padding where you can't see it. Stuffed furniture or bedding in basements is another likely place to find molds and mildew. Although we generally think of molds as growing on uphol-stered furniture, molds and mildews can also grow on wood furniture, since wood tends to absorb moisture. Molds may also grow inside the walls, or on plasterboard if there is any dampness inside the walls. If the basement has been previously flooded, molds can remain indefinitely.

If you are sensitive to molds, it is generally better not to carpet or store furniture in your basement. If possible, it is also usually a good idea to locate your washer and dryer on an upper floor, since molds thrive under such appliances and in the pipes that lead to them since that environment is often warm and damp. A dehumidifier may also be helpful in reducing the amount of mold in a damp basement.

HOUSEPLANTS. Molds often grown in the soil of indoor plants, so if you are sensitive to molds you may want to consider getting rid of your houseplants.

CLOSETS. Because many people keep closet doors closed most of the time, closets tend to be hotter than the rest of the house and also get less air circulation. Therefore, they tend to be ideal places for molds to grow. If possible, avoid jamming closets to capacity and use plastic-coated wire shelving that lets the air circulate. It also might not be a bad idea to leave closet doors open most of the time.

Shoes are particularly good places for molds to grow, especially if they are placed in closed closets while they are damp. If possible, don't put wet or damp shoes away in a closet. And frequently check shoes you don't wear very often for signs of molds.

AIR CONDITIONERS, VAPORIZERS, FURNACE FILTERS, AND HUMIDI-FIERS. Air-conditioning ducts are ideal places for molds to grow, since water may condense inside them and sit stagnant. If you are concerned about a mold problem, the air-conditioning vents in your home should be inspected and cleaned frequently. You should also be diligent about changing furnace filters and cleaning humidifiers and vaporizers, since all three may not only produce mold, but circulate it throughout your house, as well.

As discussed previously, humidity is generally good for someone with chronic nasal and sinus complaints. However, high humidity also provides an ideal climate for molds that can make chronic sinus problems worse. Thus, those with rhinosinusitis often find themselves in a catch-22 situation.

While there is no ideal solution to this problem, the best course is to use humidification, but avoid leaving it on high for a prolonged basis in order to avoid developing molds.

OUTSIDE THE HOUSE. Molds are also somewhat seasonal. For example, molds are much more prevalent in the fall, when they grow on dead leaves and branches of trees. In addition, mold accumulates in gutters, downspouts, and drains. If you have rhinosinusitis, have someone clean these out frequently, particularly in the fall when they fill with leaves (it is not wise to do it yourself in this situation).

Products that Eliminate Mold

Although there are many products on the market that claim to help eliminate mold, in most cases, household bleach will work just as well. Since bleach contains chlorine and releases chlorine gas into the atmosphere, you should use always use a diluted solution of bleach (one part bleach to ten parts water) and, when you do, either use it in a well-ventilated place or wear a respirator when applying it.

Occasionally, mold growth in the walls of buildings becomes a problem for those who are sensitive to it. Within the past few years, hundreds of lawsuits have been filed against employers and contractors by those who have claimed injury caused by what have become known as "toxic molds." Not surprisingly, a large industry has sprung up devoted to eradicating mold from homes and office buildings. Most people involved in this business are ethical, but some are not. Because mold eradication is a very expensive process, it is important that you (a) be sure that you actually have mold in your house, (b) that it is causing your rhinosinusitis symptoms, and (c) that you are dealing with a reputable mold-elimination company if you wish to have your home or business inspected or treated for mold.

Allergies

As we have discussed in several previous chapters, those who have respiratory allergies nearly always also suffer from rhinosinusitis. While it is certainly possible for people to be allergic to just about anything, the most common allergies are plant pollen, mites, animals, insects, drugs, and various foods. Some of these things are obviously much easier to stay away from than others.

FOODS AND DRUGS. If you know you are allergic to certain foods, it is usually easy to simply avoid eating them. However, since so many of today's prepared foods contain many different foods and preservatives, if you have food allergies, you need to be very diligent about reading food labels.

It is also a good idea to avoid foods that appear to cause nasal congestion, even if you are not known to be allergic to them. Nasal congestion decreases mucus clearance by the cilia and may predispose you to further inflammation. People with chronic rhinosinusitis often notice that wine (particularly red wine) and alcohol (particularly the darker alcohols) cause nasal stuffiness. It is not clear whether this is really an allergy or whether the alcohol causes dilatation of the inflamed blood vessels. However, in either case, it is strongly advisable to avoid this additional cause of nasal congestion.

If you are allergic to drugs such as penicillin, you should make sure that your doctor knows this. Another option is to wear a medical alert bracelet or necklace that can be purchased at any pharmacy. In case of an accident, hospital emergency personnel would see this alert and know not to give you penicillin.

POLLENS. While it may be comparatively easy to avoid foods and drugs to which you are allergic, other kinds of irritants are more difficult to avoid, particularly pollen. Although the actual pollen count tends to be higher in the countryside, generally, symptoms caused by pollen tend to be worse in polluted cities.

It is possible for an allergy specialist to determine exactly which pollen is causing the symptoms of your allergy but, in most cases, even if you know exactly which pollen it is, it will still be virtually impossible for you to avoid such airborne pollen. You simply need to be aware of pollen counts in your area, and be especially prepared with medications and remedies such as nasal sprays when the counts are high. The use of both chromolyn sodium (available over-the-counter as Nasalcrom) and antihistamines will be helpful during an allergy season, if you are going to spend time outside. Topical nasal steriods used on a regular basis are also very helpful.

ANIMAL DANDER. Animal dander is also a frequent cause of allergic symptoms. Obviously, the best solution for this problem is to avoid owning a pet and to avoid places where pets live. Again, however, if you live around people, you are probably likely to also live around pets of some kind or another. If you know that you are going to be around animals, your best option is probably to ask your doctor what medications you could take before contact with animals to avoid allergy symptoms.

It is important to realize that it can take many years to rid your home of pet dander after a pet has been removed from the home. Sometimes people get rid of a pet, notice no improvement after a few

months, and then buy another pet. This is a significant misunder-
standing, because the dander can remain around and cause problems
for many years after the pets have gone. If you have a pet allergy and
are not willing to keep the pet out of the house, it is important to at
least keep the pet out of the bedroom.

Sometimes, when an animal allergy is determined as a result of
allergy testing, a patient will point out that they no longer react to the
cat or dog with the same acute allergic reaction that they used to have
and will argue in favor of keeping the animal in question. Unfortunately, the lack of an acute allergic reaction does not indicate that a
pet is not still causing the problem. As people get older, allergic reactions do not have the typical acute reaction with sneezing or watery
eyes and nose, nor do they have the rapid onset of nasal obstruction
that occurred when the person was younger. Rather, the allergic
reactions simply become subtler and are characterized by a gradually
increasing nasal obstruction and, as a result, people with animal allergies begin to react to many more irritants in the environment, often
feeling that they are becoming "allergic to everything." It appears that
the allergies may "prime" them for nonspecific reactions to multiple
factors, even if they are not allergic to them. It is not known whether
staying in contact with an allergen continues this priming process, but
there is significant reason for concern that it may indeed make symptoms worse over time.

HOUSEHOLD DUST. If household dust is a problem, it may be a good
idea to install an electrostatic air filter on your furnace. While such filters can't eliminate all dust, they can still help. Many people who are
allergic to household dust find it useful to get rid of items in the house
that tend to collect dust, such as carpeting, and to dust their houses
frequently using a damp cloth to avoid stirring up dust particles.

Tips for Controlling Your Environment

The American Academy of Otolaryngology—Head and Neck Surgery recommends the following tips for controlling your environment if you are subject to allergies.

1. Wear a pollen mask when mowing grass or house cleaning (most drug and hardware stores sell them).
2. Keep windows and doors closed during heavy pollen seasons.
3. Rid your home of indoor plants and other sources of mildew.
4. Don't allow dander-producing animals into your home.
5. Replace feather pillows, woolen blankets and clothing with cotton or synthetic materials.
6. Enclose mattresses, box springs, and pillows in plastic barrier clothes.
7. Use antihistamines and decongestants as necessary and as tolerated.
8. Sleep with a brick or two placed under bedposts at the head of the bed to elevated your head to relieve nasal congestion.
9. Observe good general health practices; exercise daily, stop smoking, avoid air pollutants, eat a balanced diet, and supplement your diet with vitamins, especially vitamin C.
10. Consider using a humidifier or vaporizer in the winter. Dry, indoor heat aggravates many allergic people. Be sure to clean the humidifier regularly.

Allergy Testing and Allergy Densensitization (Allergy Shots)

If you seem to have allergies, the things that you are allergic to can be defined by allergy testing. Allergy testing can be performed either by a blood test or by small skin pricks of the allergens. Knowing the irritants that you are allergic to may help you to avoid them. This is important not just because of the discomfort that occurs when you have allergy symptoms, but also because, if you continue to have allergy exposure and allergy symptoms over time, it can make the chronic symptoms of rhinosinusitis and asthma worse, even in the absence of acute allergy symptoms. If you have allergies that you cannot avoid and that are not well controlled with anti-histamines or topical nasal steroids, your doctor may suggest allergy densensitization.

Things to Avoid

In addition to the precautions discussed earlier in this chapter, if you are subject to rhinosinusitis, it is probably also a good idea to avoid the items described below.

THINGS THAT DRY OUT THE MUCOUS MEMBRANES. Many things dry out the mucous membranes, but the most common are dry indoor heat in the winter, alcoholic beverages, and a number of medications such as diuretics and anti-anxiety medication.

THINGS THAT INTERFERE WITH THE FUNCTION OF THE CILIA. If the cilia (the tiny hairs that circulate mucus) cannot work, mucus will thicken, back up into the nasal passage and sinuses, and an infection can occur. Tobacco or marijuana smoke are two of the major culprits in paralyzing cilia. Overuse or incorrect use of nasal sprays or irrigations can also damage the cilia.

THINGS THAT CAUSE THE NASAL MEMBRANES TO SWELL. Swelling in the nasal membranes can be caused by many things. Infections cause swelling, as do airborne irritants to which people are allergic. Nasal membranes can also swell during pregnancy or as a result of the menstrual cycle. Some medications, including leukotrine modifiers used to treat asthma and some allergies, some antidepressants, some blood pressure medications and overuse of decongestants can also be the culprits, as can caffeine, alcoholic beverages, and food allergies. In order to avoid this uncomfortable situation, you need to work with your doctor to figure out what the causes of the swelling in your sinuses may be.

SWIMMING. Swimming pools are treated with chlorine, which can irritate the lining of the nose and sinuses. In addition, public swimming pools and bathhouses provide excellent places for molds and bacteria to grow. While the purpose of chlorine in the water of public pools is to kill bacteria and molds, if pool chemicals are not properly used, and with that many people in one place, bacteria are likely to spread quickly from person to person. Additionally, the chlorine itself can be very irritating to someone who has rhinosinusitis and hyperreactive mucosa in their nose. Although fewer people are likely to be around, swimming in a lake, river, or pond has its own hazards for those who are subject to rhinosinusitis. Unchlorinated freshwater may be full of bacteria, molds, fungi, and a host of pollutants. Swimming in nonpolluted ocean water (if you can find it) will actually wash out the nose and sinuses and can be helpful. If you enjoy swimming, check with your doctor to see what your best course of action should be.

SCUBA DIVING. Scuba divers typically choose clean, clear, nonpolluted areas to practice their sport so, for those people with sinusitis, salt water diving can provide an effective nasal and sinus wash. However, people with nasal allergies, nasal congestion, and chronic rhinosinusitis frequently have trouble with the pressure changes associated with diving, either with pain in the sinuses (a sinus squeeze) or in ears (ear squeeze). Because the pressure changes are so marked in diving, it is essential that, if someone starts to get a "squeeze", they ascend enough to release the feeling of pressure and then try to equalize their ears. Failure to do this can result in permanent damage, most frequently to the ears, but also occasionally to the sinuses. The pressure changes with a sinus obstruction during diving can actually strip the lining mucosa off the bone and cause permanent changes. Of course, it is dangerous to dive with a cold or with acute allergies. If you enjoy diving and do not have acute congestion, you may just have to see what effect, if any, it has on you.

AIR TRAVEL. As with diving, air travel causes pressure changes in the sinuses and ears, which need to be equalized by air going in or out of the sinuses or Eustachian tubes. However, the pressure changes are not as great or as rapid as they are with diving. Typically, the greater problem is on airplane descent, when the cabin pressure increases and air needs to enter these spaces. If the air does not enter, the pain can be intense. Small children have less well-developed Eustachian tubes than adults and do not know to swallow or chew to equalize the pressure in their ears and are therefore more prone to ear pain. This is why you may have noticed that so many babies cry during descent. Small babies can be helped by feeding or by sucking on a pacifier. The movement of their palate will help to open the Eustachian tubes and improve the chances of equalization. This remedy needs to be started as soon as the plane starts to descend, before the ears become "locked" by a significant pressure differential.

However, these maneuvers will not help the sinuses. Because of this, and because flying with a cold significantly increases the risk of developing a bacterial rhinosinutis, it is wise not to fly when you have a cold. Flying may also exacerbate chronic rhinosinusitis or precipitate sinusitis in the absence of a cold. The reason for this is unclear, but the pressure changes, as well as the very dry recirculated air in the cabin and even fatigue and jet lag, may all be partial factors.

Rhinosinusitis sufferers can lessen the symptoms and problems associated with flying by:

1. taking an oral decongestant prior to the flight.
2. using normal saline sprays during the flight.
3. using a topical decongestant spray a half hour prior to descent.
4. beginning topical nasal steroids several days prior to the flight.

Those who frequently experience severe symptoms may occasionally need to take prescription oral steroid medications for a couple of days before and after the flight, although oral steroids also have their own risks.

OVERUSE OF ANTIBIOTICS. In Chapter 11, we discussed in some detail the problems that have developed because of the overuse of antibiotics, the main issue being the development of antibiotic resistance. Because so many rhinosinusitis infections are bacterial in nature, antibiotics are still often the best possible treatment for them. But in order for them to be effective, it is important that you not have taken so many of them that it is difficult to find one that still works for the bacteria that you now have in your nose. For this reason, before prescribing an antibiotic, your doctor may well suggest that you try one of the therapies discussed in chapter 10. If you are subject to chronic rhinosinusitis, your doctor may also suggest that you consider surgery.

MISUSE OF OVER-THE-COUNTER MEDICATIONS. Many over-the-counter medications (medications that do not require a prescription) can be very effective in treating the symptoms of rhinosinusitis, although, of course, they cannot cure infections. There are also several other factors to consider when taking an over-the-counter medication.

1. Many over-the-counter remedies contain not just one, but several medications such as a decongestant, analgesic, and expectorant. In some cases, you may benefit from all of these medications but, in other cases, one of the ingredients in these combination products may actually make your symptoms worse.

2. Taking any medication for a long period of time can often have what is known as the "rebound effect." This occurs when a medication no longer works for a patient and taking the drug actually makes the symptoms recur or get worse. This effect is a particular problem with topical nasal decongestant sprays.

3. Some medications, particularly nasal sprays, if overused, can actually damage the mucous membranes, inflame the tissue, and cause an infection to develop.

4. In many cases, it is a good idea to treat the symptoms of a disease; in other cases continuing to treat symptoms masks the actual underlying cause of the disease. If you feel that you need to constantly take an over-the-counter medication, it is a good idea to see a doctor to see if another course of treatment might be better for you.

Beware of Using Herbal Remedies or Alternative Therapies

As we discussed in Chapter 15, many herbal remedies and alternative therapies can help relieve sinusitis symptoms. Unfortunately, their effects can also be unpredictable, because they are not subject to approval by the FDA. Many such products are imported from other countries, and there is no way to ensure what the contents, purity, strength, or efficacy of these products really is, because their effectiveness has not been scientifically proven. Before using these remedies or therapies, ask your doctor's opinion.

TAKE CARE OF YOUR NOSE. Because most of the contaminants that cause rhinosinusitis enter the body through the nose, you must be especially diligent about paying attention to the following list of tips.

1. Always avoid blowing your nose forcefully, or with both nostrils at the same time. Instead, block one nostril and gently blow on one side at a time.

2. Drink plenty of fluids to keep the mucus hydrated.
3. Use nasal decongestant or saline sprays wisely. Remember that topical decongestant sprays should never be used for more than three to five days. Correct use of these products can greatly relieve your symptoms, but overuse or misuse can make your condition worse.
4. Before you use these products, it is a good idea to ask your doctor or pharmacist how to use them correctly.

How to Prevent Your Rhinosinusitis from Getting Worse

Although you may not always be able to prevent an attack of sinusitis, there are several things that you can do to keep your sinusitis from getting worse.

1. Increase your water intake.
2. Use nasal rinses, humidifiers, steam, and saline nasal sprays.
3. Avoid excessive forceful nose blowing.
4. Stop smoking and stay away from people who are smoking. Smoking irritates the lining of your nose, whether you are smoking or others around you are smoking. Obviously, the situation is worse if you are the one who is smoking.
5. Consult a doctor if you find that you have developed thick yellow or green mucus, have increasing discomfort, or your symptoms are not improving within a week.

17

THE COST
OF SINUSITIS
Treatment and Insurance Factors

NOTHING MAY BE MORE FRUSTRATING FOR A consumer today than trying to figure out how the health care insurance system really works, and what may or may not be covered for treatment of any disease, including sinusitis. There are literally hundreds of different options available and, among these options, costs vary considerably from one region of the county to another. In general, most health care services are more expensive in urban centers and on the coasts than they are in small towns and in the Midwest and mountain states, but there are always exceptions.

While it will not be possible to give you specific information when it comes to how much it will cost to treat your rhinosinusitis, this chapter should give you a general idea of what some medications cost. It will also provide an overview of how the insurance system works in this country and suggest questions you should ask your doctor as you work together to decide what type of treatment may be the best for you.

Health Insurance

It probably goes without saying that you really should have at least some health insurance, regardless of whether you are single or have a family. Even the most basic health care can be quite expensive and, if you don't have health insurance, many health care providers will not treat you or will insist that you pay for your health care service at the time the service is provided.

Health insurance today is often provided as part of an employee's benefits package. However, as the cost of health insurance rises, employers are increasingly expecting their employees to assume part of the cost with higher annual contributions and copayments. People who are self-employed or who work for companies that do not provide health insurance benefits often purchase such insurance through an association or other organization in order to take advantage of the group rates provided. In any case, such insurance is known as private health insurance, because it is not managed by the government. The following are some of the most common kinds of nongovernmental health insurance.

PRIVATE HEALTH INSURANCE. If your employer includes health care insurance in your benefits package, chances are that coverage is structured in one of three ways: (1) an indemnity plan, (2) a preferred provider organization (PPO), or (3) a health maintenance organization (HMO). If your company has an employee handbook, details about your health insurance should be included. If you don't have an employee handbook, your human resources department or the person in charge of hiring employees should be able to give you this information.

INDEMNITY PLANS. If your employer has an indemnity insurance plan, generally that means that you may choose your own physician, hospital, and place where you buy your medications. Most employers that have indemnity plans issue their employees an identification card, which usually looks like a credit card and has a magnetic strip on the back that can be scanned by service providers. When you use one of these services, the physician, hospital, or pharmacy will bill you and/or your employer in one of four ways.

1. The bill for this service will be submitted to your employer (or directly to your employer's insurance carrier), and the employer will pay all of the costs of this service.

2. Your employer will pay a part of the costs and require that you pay the difference between what the doctor, hospital, or pharmacy charges and what your employer will pay. This type of plan is sometimes called a "co-pay."

3. You will be required to pay the total cost of the service or medication, then submit your receipts and your employer will reimburse you.

4. You will be required to pay your portion of the bill at the time of your office visit, hospital stay, or prescription purchase and they (the doctor, hospital, or pharmacy) will bill the employer's portion directly to the employer.

PREFERRED PROVIDER ORGANIZATIONS. Preferred provider organizations (PPOs) are groups of physicians and/or hospitals that have an agreement with local employers that provide discounts on services if the employers agree to use their services exclusively. If your employer has an agreement with a PPO, then you, as an employee, will be given a list of physicians and hospitals from which to choose. When you have an office visit or a hospital stay, the payment procedure will be the same as if you had an indemnity plan (see above). You will often have to pay a small co-payment, usually ranging from $10 to $25 per visit.

Health Maintenance Organizations

Your employer may have an agreement with an HMO which differs from PPOs in that an HMO is often a physical facility with a staff of

either primary care providers or primary care providers and specialists. Some HMOs also run hospitals and pharmacies, as well. If this is
the case, you will be required to use this facility and this staff of doctors. In some cases, you may be able to choose a physician from the
HMO staff, and you will see that physician for all of your visits. In
other cases, a physician will be assigned to you. And, in yet other
instances, when you make an appointment you may be seen by whatever doctor is working at the HMO at that time.

Usually an employer who has an HMO plan will not pay for the
cost of visiting a specialist, such as an otolaryngologist, unless that
specialist is on the staff of the HMO or you are referred to the specialist by the primary care physician at the HMO. As with indemnity
plans or PPOs, whether you pay a portion of the costs of this service
and how you pay it will depend on what kind of arrangement you or
your employer has with the HMO. Again, a co-payment is usually
charged at the time of service.

Government Health Insurance

MEDICARE. Medicare is a federal health care program that was created in 1965 by the US Department of Heath and Human Services
(formerly the Department of Health, Education, and Welfare) to help
ensure that older Americans have access to affordable health care. In
1972, the program was expanded to include people with disabilities
and end-stage renal disease.

Medicare is divided into two plans, A and B. Plan A is hospital
insurance and Plan B is insurance that covers other costs, such as doctor office visits. If you are older than 65 and you and/or your spouse
have worked outside the home and paid Medicare taxes for at least 10
years, you are eligible to receive Part A at no additional cost to you.
(If you and/or your spouse have not worked outside the home and
paid Medicare taxes for 10 years, you may have to purchase Plan A.)
Everyone who wishes to have Plan B must purchase it. The current

cost of Plan B is $54 per month. Originally, Medicare was strictly a reimbursement plan, but now physicians and hospitals can bill Medicare directly. For more specific information about Medicare, visit the official Medicare website (www.Medicare.gov).

As with other health insurance plans, not all costs of office visits or hospital stays are covered by Medicare. So if you qualify for Medicare, you should ask your doctor what portion of your treatment is covered and what you should expect to pay. In most states, the cost of prescription medications is not covered by Medicare except those medications received during a hospital stay.

In August 2002, the federal government began an experimental program that offers 11 million Medicare participants in 23 states the option to use PPOs. (It also allows participants to choose physicians outside the PPO network if they agree to pay extra.) This is the first time that prescription drugs will be paid for by Medicare when a patient is not in the hospital.

MEDIGAP INSURANCE. Because, until 2003, Medicare did not pay for prescription medications except those used in the hospital, or 100% of all health care costs, many people purchased a Medigap health insurance policy (and must continue to do so in those states not included in the experimental plan). While Medigap policies supplement Medicare, they are not affiliated with or regulated by the federal government. There are now many Medigap policies available and they offer different benefits. The cost of Medigap policies varies considerably, so you should always shop around before purchasing such a policy. The American Association of Retired Persons (AARP) has a lot of important information about Medigap Insurance, and will provide that information to you free of charge. You can reach AARP at www.AARP.org., call them at 1-800-424-3410, or write to them at 601 E St. NW, Washington, DC, 20049.

MEDICAID. Medicare was created to provide older working Americans with affordable health care. Medicaid was created to help the indigent. Medicaid is a combination state and federal program so qualifications vary from state to state. Medicaid generally pays all or at least most of the cost of office visits, hospital stays, and medication, but the regulations involving that care are generally more stringent that those for Medicare recipients. Usually, to receive Medicaid a person must be sufficiently indigent to qualify for a state's welfare program. To find out if you qualify for Medicaid, you can visit the official Medicaid website (www.cms.hhs.gov), or call the agency in your community that provides welfare benefits.

HOW HEALTH CARE COSTS ARE DETERMINED. Unlike countries such as Canada or Sweden, the United States does not have a federally subsidized health care system (other than Medicare and Medicaid), so theoretically, at least, physicians, hospitals, and pharmaceutical companies can charge whatever they want to for their services. However, since most patients and employers have choices about what they will pay for, most health care providers determine prices for products and services based on what Diagnosis Related Group (DRG) the service or procedure falls within. DRGs were created in 1983 to help contain Medicare costs in hospitals but, since that time, they have also been used by private insurers, as well, to try to determine what the "usual and customary" costs of any particular procedure should be. There are now 503 possible classifications of diagnoses in the DRG listings, so most physicians and hospitals can generally find one that fits the situation faced by a particular patient.

Again, because the U.S. health care system is not controlled by the government, physicians and hospitals are free to charge whatever they want to, but most private insurance companies and/or employers as well as federal insurance providers such as Medicare and Medicaid will only pay the costs estimated by the DRGs.

THE COST OF MEDICAL TESTS. As with office visits and hospital stays, the costs of medical tests are generally determined by what DRG they fall within, although these costs may also vary by geographical location or whether the tests are performed in a large city. Thanks to computer technology, many diagnostic tests can now be performed right in the doctor's office and results given to the patient within a few minutes. Other diagnostic tests are performed either at an independent laboratory or testing facility. As with all other medical services, the private insurer, Medicare, or Medicaid may require that tests be performed at a specific location by a specific provider. Before you have a diagnostic test performed, you should ask both your doctor and your insurance carrier what the cost of such a test will be and where it may be performed. Only then can you determine what the cost to you will be.

THE COST OF SURGERY. A system has also been created to help standardize the costs of surgical procedures. Although diagnostic coding was done as early as the seventeenth century in England, it wasn't until the late 1940s that the World Health Organization (WHO) published the International Classification of Diseases (ICD). In 1988, a provision of the Medicare Catastrophic Coverage Act required that each Medicare Part B claim include the appropriate ICD codes. Now, most insurers insist on the inclusion of these codes as well, when determining how much they will reimburse physicians for medical services, including surgery. Still, it is often very difficult to estimate the exact cost of a particular surgery because, in many instances, the surgeon won't know for sure what all will be involved until the surgery is underway. As with other medical services, before you have this service provided, it is a good idea to talk with both your insurance provider and your doctor to determine what the anticipated costs to you may be.

THE COST OF MEDICATIONS. Most private health care plans, Medicaid and, in some states, Medicare, cover at least a portion of the cost of prescription medications. Very few insurance plans cover the cost of over-the-counter (nonprescription) medications. Whether you have an indemnity plan, a PPO, or are part of an HMO, your employer (or some Medicare plans or Medicaid) will cover the costs of your medicines in one of several ways.

1. Cover the cost of all of your medications. (Few companies do this.)
2. Cover the total cost of some of your medications. (For example, if you work for a pharmaceutical company, the company may cover the total cost of all medications they manufacture and give you a discount on medications they don't manufacture.)
3. Charge you a fixed fee for every prescription (for example, $10) no matter what it is.
4. Share the cost of medications with you through a co-pay arrangement in which you pay a certain percentage or dollar amount for your medications.

HOW YOU OBTAIN YOUR MEDICATIONS. If you are a member of an HMO, that organization may also have a pharmacy located in the building. If so, chances are your employer will require that you get your medications at that pharmacy.

You should be aware that most HMOs and PPOs often restrict physicians' choice of medicines they can prescribe to you. In addition, your insurer may also restrict the quantity of medication your physician will be allowed to prescribe per day or month.

When choosing your insurance coverage, you should keep the prescription drug plan rules in mind, particularly if you have a known underlying ailment that will require ongoing prescription medicine.

If you are part of an indemnity plan, your employer may require that you get all your medications (at least the medications for which they are paying some or all of the cost) at a specific pharmacy. In some cases, the employer may require that you order your prescription medications from a mail-order or Internet-based pharmacy.

BRAND NAMES VERSUS GENERICS. Some medications have no generic equivalents because the pharmaceutical company that developed the medication still holds the patent to the medication. If the patent on a medication has expired, generic versions are probably available. Some employers and health plans only pay for the generic medication. While there is some ongoing debate about whether the generic versions of medications are as effective as the originals, because they are pharmacologically similar, the end effect should be about the same.

Regulations about generic medications also vary from state to state. In some states, the law requires that a pharmacist offer you the option of purchasing the generic version of the medication. In other states, the pharmacist may simply substitute the generic version of the medication for what the physician prescribed and not tell the patient. In yet other states, the pharmacist may even substitute an entirely different medication from the one your doctor prescribed.

Before you have a prescription filled, you should check with your doctor to see what the law is in your state, and whether or not your doctor feels you should have the brand-name medication or whether a generic will work just as well.

AVERAGE COSTS OF SINUSITIS MEDICATIONS. Again, the costs of all medications can vary greatly, depending on where you purchase them, how they are purchased, and how your insurer or employer reimburses you. To give you a general idea of the cost of a few sinusitis medications, the following chart reflects what each medication would cost if you paid full price for it at a Midwestern grocery store pharmacy chain in 2004.

Prices of Over-the-Counter Sinusitis Medications

Nonprescription Medication	Form	Quantity	Full Cost *(in dollars and cents)*
Irrigated Mists			
Entsol®	adapter; nasal wash tip with comfort release valve	1	28.99
Entsol®	mist; buffered hypertonic nasal irrigation mist	1 fl. Oz	54.99
Entsol®	packets; powdered buffered hypertonic nasal wash	10 each	6.99
Entsol®	refillable, reusable nasal wash squeeze bottle	1	29.99
Entsol®	single use, prefilled nasal wash squeeze bottle	1	5.99
Entsol®	spray, buffered hypertonic saline nasal spray	100 ml	14.99
WaterPik®	professional oral irrigator	1	54.99
Decongestants			
Afrin®	12-hour decongestant nasal spray	5 fl. oz.	5.49
Benzedrex Inhaler®	propylhexedrine nasal decongestant	1	5.29
Comtrex®	maximum strength sinus and nasal decongestant	20	5.99
Dristan®	12-hour decongestant nasal spray	5 fl. oz.	6.29
4-Way®	fast-acting nasal decongestant spray	1 oz.	6.99
Neo-Synephrine®	12-hour decongestant spray	5 fl. Oz.	4.99
Sudafed®	12-hour non-drowsy nasal decongestant coated tablets	14	4.49
Vicks®	vapor inhaler	.01 oz	3.49
Allergy			
Claritin®	12-hour tablets	10	12.00
Claritin®	24-hour tablets	20	17.99
Combination Products			
Aleve®	cold and sinus caplets, pain reliever/ fever reducer/nasal decongestant	20	7.99
Congestac®	nasal decongestant-expectorant	24	8.59
Ornex®	maximum strength nasal decongestant and analgesic	24	7.89
Robitussin®	nasal decongestant and expectorant	8 fl. oz.	6.99
Vapor Rubs			
Vicks Vapo Rub®	nasal decongestant and cough suppressant cream	2 oz.	4.49

PRICES OF PRESCRIPTION ANTIBIOTICS

Amoxil®	250 mg	30	17.00
Augmentin®	250 mg	30	85.00
Avelox®	400 mg	30	240.00
Biaxin®	250 mg	30	120.00
Cedax®	400 mg	30	220.00
Ceftin®	125 mg	30	65.00
Cipro®	500 mg	14	190.00
Doryx®	100 mg	30	85.00
Levaquin®	250 mg	24	490.00
Lorabid®	200 mg	30	133.00
Suprax®		14	57.99
Vantin®	100 mg	14	48.99
Zithromax®	250 mg	24	159.00
Tequin®	200 mg	30	275.00

The American Association of Retired Persons (AARP) has produced a pamphlet, "Drug Smart", that offers suggestions on the various ways prescriptions may be filled and a guide to obtaining the best value for your prescription dollar. To obtain this pamphlet, you may call 1-800-424-3410, write to AARP at 601 E St. NW, Washington, D.C. 20049, or visit www.modernmaturity.org.

18

SPECIAL CASES

Children, Those with Cystic Fibrosis, and More

LTHOUGH ANYBODY CAN GET SINUSITIS, AND, as we discussed in Chapter 1, more than 37 million Americans suffer from at least one acute attack per year, some people are much more likely than others to contract the disease. Among these are children, pregnant women, the elderly, immune-suppressed patients, and those people who have some specific rare diseases or conditions.

Children

Because the sinuses are not completely formed until around age 20, children and teenagers are more prone to infections of the nose, sinuses, and ears than older children and adults. They also get more colds each year.

By far the most common causes of rhinosinusitis in children are the common cold and other viral infections.

Chronic sinusitis may also present in children with a nighttime cough, a symptom that is not commonly seen in adults.

TREATMENT. Even very young children can be treated in the same way as older children or adults. Many antibiotics can be safely given to small children. However, tetracyclines and the quinolone group of antibiotics (Cipro®, Levaquin®, Avelox®, and so forth) should be avoided. Quinolones should not be given to children because of a chance of damage to cartilage and joint development. Tetracycline is contraindicated for children under the age of 8 because it can cause permanent discoloration of the teeth.

Topical nasal decongestants and oral decongestants may also help alleviate symptoms. In chronic rhinosinusitis and severe nasal allergies, a number of the topical nasal steroids may also be used in children and, when the problems are marked, the benefits outweigh the risks. Studies have shown that topical nasal steroids can, at least initially, cause some slowing of the normal growth curve. However, children appear to catch up later, even if the topical steroid is continued. Because it is very important that children be given an appropriate dosage (usually determined by the child's weight), it is essential to consult the child's doctor before using any medication.

Pregnant Women

During pregnancy, many women experience rhinitis of pregnancy, an inflammation of the nasal lining that blocks mucus drainage. Because this condition is thought to be caused by hormonal changes, it may also occur in women who take birth control pills. Although rhinitis of pregnancy may have the same symptoms as a sinus infection, an infection is often not present, and antibiotics are not needed to relieve symptoms.

TREATMENT. Because it is problematic to take medications during pregnancy, it is generally recommended that pregnant women relieve the inflammation through the use of saltwater nasal sprays or over-the-counter decongestant sprays. If an infection does occur, some antibiotics may be safely prescribed. In any event, it is always important that a pregnant woman check with a doctor before taking any kind of medication.

The Elderly

As with most parts of the body, the nose changes with age. Typically, as a person ages, the tip of the nose begins to droop, causing the nose to narrow and elongate and decreasing the amount of space through which air can flow. In some cases, the cartilage in the nose thins and softens. The mucus-secreting structures in the nose gradually atrophy, resulting in decreased mucus production and nasal dryness. Because of this dryness, elderly people are more likely to have nosebleeds than younger people. Older people also often feel a chronic need to clear the throat, especially when they lie down. In some cases, medications such as Evista, Fosamax, and Miacalcin used to treat osteoporosis can cause rhinosinusitis symptoms.

Because elderly people tend to suffer from more than one chronic illness, they may be taking several medications. As we discussed in Chapter 11, rhinitis and rhinosinusitis are side effects of many medications, so those who take several medications are more likely to develop rhinosinusitis from one of them.

The elderly may also develop rhinosinusitis from dental infections or other types of respiratory infections. One particular problem that appears to occur almost exclusively in the elderly is the problem of a persistently drippy nose. The reason for this watery discharge is not known.

Fortunately, as a person ages, most problems with allergies tend to diminish, so the elderly are generally less bothered with seasonal rhinitis than younger people.

TREATMENT. When the problem is primarily nasal obstruction at night, use of a plastic strip on the nose at night can help hold the nasal passages open. In severe cases of nasal obstruction due to softening of the cartilage, nasal surgery may be recommended.

Because dryness is such a factor, older people may also benefit from inhaling steam, using a saline wash, and drinking six to eight glasses of water a day. If infection develops, antibiotics may be prescribed but, since the metabolism of older people is different from that of younger people, it is important that the doctor give the appropriate dosage.

If the problem is a drippy nose, some patients may be helped by taking a proton pump inhibitor (for example, Nexium®, Protonix®, Prevacid®), medications normally prescribed for the treatment of heartburn. These are prescription medications, but if a drippy nose is a significant problem, it is worth discussing it with your physician. Atrovent® nasal spray is another medication that is sometimes helpful in this situation.

People with Cystic Fibrosis

Chronic rhinosinusitis and nasal polyps are extremely common in people with cystic fibrosis (CF), a congenital disorder that results in the secretion of large amounts of thickened mucus that clogs the lungs and upper respiratory system. Generally, those with CF develop rhinosinusitis sometime between the ages of 5 and 14, but there is considerable variation in the time of onset. In fact, in recent years, we have learned that the only symptom of milder variations of CF may be sinusitis. As a result, we recommend that everyone who has sinus disease serious enough to require sinus surgery before the age of 20 undergo testing for CF. Today, this can be performed with a simple genetic blood test. As with all genetic tests, it is important to consider the advantages and disadvantages of the test before it is performed.

While chronic rhinosinusitis is uncomfortable for anyone who has it, in a person with CF it can be more severe and more serious. The tendency to form and reform polyps is much greater in a person with

CF, and it is very difficult to keep the polyps under control, even with the best combination of medical therapy and surgery. In addition, CF patients with chronic sinusitis face an even greater threat of contracting pneumonia than most people, and it is possible for those with persistent sinusitis to have a recurrence of pulmonary disease even following a procedure such as a lung transplant. Although it is very difficult to control sinus disease when a patient has CF, it is important that it is managed as well as possible, so as to minimize the risk of causing further damage to the lungs.

TREATMENT. Because rhinosinusitis tends to be chronic in people with CF, endoscopic surgery (described in Chapter 13) is often the best treatment. If the surgery is successful, the airways are reopened and the risk of subsequent infection is reduced. However, over time, repeated surgery may be required. It is often recommended that patients with CF frequently irrigate the sinuses, and the use of an antiobiotic irrigation may be helpful. Those with CF may also find relief from symptoms by using nasal steroids and decongestants.

Hospitalized Patients

People who are hospitalized are at higher risk than the general population for contracting rhinosinusitis, particularly if they have suffered a head injury, are taking antibiotics or steroids, have a condition that requires insertion of tubes in the nose, or are using ventilators. Typically, however, sinusitis caused by a tube in the nose will disappear when the offending tube is removed.

People with HIV/AIDS or Other Immunologically Compromised Patients

When the immune system of the body is compromised (weakened by HIV/AIDS or other diseases, for example, chemotherapy or drugs that prevent rejection of a transplanted organ), it is often unable to fight off even the least serious diseases. Thus, it is not surprising that people with compromised immune systems often get rhinosinusitis.

Because of the potential that these infections will spread in someone who has a compromised immune system, an aggressive management of these infections is recommended. Additionally, people with compromised immune systems will sometimes get infections from unusual bacteria that do not normally cause a problem in people with normal immune systems. Taking cultures directly from the site of infection is therefore recommended; the antibiotic therapy is then based both upon the culture and antibiotic-sensitivity results.

Although most fungal sinusitis occurs in patients with normal immune systems, we are very concerned when fungal sinusitis occurs in someone who is immunosuppressed. In this situation, the fungus can rapidly spread into the tissues and cause a life-threatening problem.

TREATMENT. Bacterial sinusitis in patients who are immunosuppressed requires more aggressive therapy. This means that we are more likely to prescribe antibiotics to patients with a suspected bacterial sinusitis. However, for milder sinus symptoms, we recommend using humidification, steam, and topical nasal steroid sprays.

When an immunosuppressed patient has fungal sinusitis, it might require aggressive action involving surgery and/or intravenous antifungal therapy.

Sarcoidosis

Sarcoidosis is an uncommon disease in which small nodules occur in the lungs, the skin and, less commonly, in the lining of the nose. The underlying cause of this disease is not known, but it has been suggested that it is an unusual immunologic reaction to a bacteria. Although the primary symptoms associated with sarcoidosis occur in the lung, these "granulomas" can cause nasal obstruction when they occur in the nose and the sinuses, and give rise to chronic sinusitis. The diagnosis of sarcoidosis is made by biopsy of one of the lesions.

TREATMENT. The primary treatment of sarcoidosis is with steroids to reduce the immunological reaction. When the disease occurs intranasally, it can sometimes be managed with topical or injected steroids, but often prolonged courses of oral steroids are required. Endoscopic sinus surgery can sometimes be helpful in providing sinus drainage and reducing the level of inflammation, but such surgery does not resolve the underlying cause of the problem. One of the major problems with this disorder is that scarring usually increases. Accordingly, if surgery is performed, it is very important for the patient to take an adequate course of oral steroids in the correct dosage to ensure that scarring following the surgery is minimized and that careful postoperative endoscopic follow-up is performed.

Kartagener's Syndrome

Kartagener's Syndrome is a rare genetic disease that combines three major symptoms: chronic enlargement of the bronchial tubes (bronchiectasis), sinusitis, and situs inversus, in which the major organs of the body are in reversed position from normal. For reasons that are not well understood, the cilia (tiny hairs on the cells that move mucus along) do not function in those with Kartagener's Syndrome.

TREATMENT. Because the cilia are not working, it is difficult to clear the secretions from the sinuses, and the retained secretions will be at risk of becoming bacterially infected. Creating openings into the sinuses to allow them to drain by gravity may be of some help in this situation, as may antibiotic nasal irrigations and nasal suction.

Wegener's Granulomatosis

Wegener's Granulomatosis is another very rare disease that causes the small blood vessels to become inflamed. Those who suffer from this disease typically develop chronic nasal congestion and sinusitis, inflammation of the kidneys, and nodules in the lungs. Crusting in the nose becomes a major problem, and nosebleeds may occur. This disease is characterized by a low nasal bridge (saddle nose), a flattening of the end of the nose, and increased nasal obstruction.

TREATMENT. The best treatment for this disease seems to be a combination of a steroid, such as Prednisone, and cytotoxic medication, such as Cytoxan, which, unfortunately, can have serious side-effects such as infertility, tumor growth, infection and bone marrow suppression.

19

FUTURE TRENDS

Treatment and Procedures Now Undergoing Trials

A S NEW DIAGNOSTIC PROCEDURES ARE DISCOVERED and advances made in the understanding of related conditions and diseases, there is always more to learn about treatments for rhinosinusitis. The following are some of the areas that are now of interest to otolaryngologists.

Newer and Better Antibiotics

As we have discussed several times in this book, although there are many types of antibiotics on the market, patient allergies and/or antibiotic resistance often make it difficult to fight infections. Therefore, we're always interested in the discovery of new types of antibiotics, or ways antibiotics can work together to cure rhinosinusitis infections. For example, one recent study of 278 patients suggests that a beta-lactamase-stable oral cephalosporin (Cefprozil) causes fewer adverse side effects such as diarrhea, nausea, and rash, than amoxicillin clavulanate augmentin.

Better Antibiotic Delivery Systems

In addition to finding newer and better antibiotics, researchers are also always looking at ways to get the antibiotics to the source of infection, so as to produce quicker and more efficacious results, with fewer side effects and reduced distress, to the patient. At present, some researchers are examining methods of applying antibiotics and other medications directly to the surface of sinuses.

One promising development is the introduction of intranasal nebulized antibiotics. This delivery system involves converting compounded medications into particles small enough to disperse within the sinus cavities, yet large enough to be deposited into the sinuses. This is accomplished by use of a mist that allows the medication to go directly into the nose. The advantage of this delivery system is that the antibiotics are not circulated through the bloodstream as they would if they were oral or intravenous antibiotics. The patient can administer the medication through a machine called a nebulizer, and the treatment takes about 20 minutes. Most physicians recommend that the treatments be done two to three times daily for three weeks.

Another interesting development is the concept of using a material that could be placed into the sinuses, that will slowly dissolve and release either antibiotics or other medications, to decrease inflammation. This approach is still in development, although hyaluron, a material approved to treat sinusitis following sinus surgery, is said to have some bioactivity in promoting healing.

Genetic Link to Cystic Fibrosis

A connection between sinusitis and CF has been recognized for a long time. However, we now know that some cases of severe chronic sinusitis, even in the absence of any other clinical evidence of CF, may be caused by changes in the same genes that cause CF or very minor manifestations of CF. Ordinarily, the gene CRTR regulates the flow of salt and water across the cell membrane. People with CF carry two copies of an altered CFTR gene, which causes them to accumulate thick, sticky mucus that is difficult to clear and provides a breeding ground for bacteria. Scientists are now studying this gene to see how common CFTR alterations are in people with chronic rhinosinusitis and how they can affect people with sinusitis who do not have CF.

An Enzyme Thought to Play an Unexpected Role in Asthma

Researchers funded by the National Institute of Allergy and Infectious Diseases have discovered sets of genes that may play a key role for the enzyme arginase in causing asthmatic symptoms. If this study proves valid, it may be possible to develop new antiasthma drugs to block arginase activity. Since asthma is known to be linked to sinusitis, this discovery could impact sinusitis research as well.

In an article published in Volume 8, No. 9 of *Pulmonary Reviews.com,* it was reported that studies had shown that, when researchers induced asthma in mice, then analyzed lung tissue to see which genes were most active following asthma attacks, they found arginase, which was previously thought to be limited to the liver. Researchers then analyzed fluid and tissue samples from the lungs of asthmatic people and compared them to tissues from non-asthmatic control subjects. No arginase was found in the control samples, but significant amounts were found in the asthmatic lungs. The conclusion was that arginase appears to be the molecule that "kicks off" the chain reaction leading to asthmatic symptoms. The hope now is to find a drug that targets arginase.

The Role of Bone in Chronic Rhinosinusitis

One of our particular areas of research interest is the role that inflammation of bone plays in chronic sinus inflammation. Bone inflammation responds very poorly to medical therapy, and both our clinical work, and our work in our laboratories at the University of Pennsylvania, have demonstrated that the bone becomes significantly involved in the inflammatory process. This has implications for how we treat patients, both medically and surgically, as well as providing one of the reasons why chronic sinusitis, when significantly advanced, is difficult to resolve. In the future, we also hope that improved understanding of this process will enable us develop medical strategies to block the bone inflammation, and thus significantly reduce the difficulty in treatment of chronic sinusitis.

The Role of Biofilms in Chronic Sinusitis

The importance of relatively small numbers of bacteria living in colonies has been studied as it relates to dental plaque. However, more recently, similar bacterial colonies have been identified in middle ear fluid in children. This has importance in managing chronic sinusitis because these bacteria are protected by a coating of mucus and are relatively impervious to antibiotics. More recently, James Palmer, MD, at the University of Pennsylvania has been evaluating this same phenomenon in sinusitis, and if our early work is confirmed, it may provide an alternative approach to this problem, using more local cleansing of the sinus mucosal surface as one of the methods to reduce the inflammatory process. Indeed, Xylitol irrigations are being used by some physicians based upon this concept.

Treating Loss of Sense of Smell

Richard Doty, at the University of Pennsylvania Smell and Taste Center, has demonstrated that the sense of smell decreases with age and that, generally, it is better in women than in men, and worse in smokers. Until recently, it was assumed that the loss of smell as a result of aging was inevitable. However, researchers Robert C.

Kern, MD, D. B. Conley, MD, G. K. Haines III, MD, and A. M. Rotinson, MD have demonstrated that apoptosis (programmed cell death) is a significant component of olfactory sensory neuron loss, raising the possibility that drugs may be developed to help to avoid this condition.

Connection with Chronic Fatigue Syndrome

The results of a study released by Georgetown University Medical Center in August, 2003, suggest that there may, in some cases, be a link between sinusitis and chronic fatigue syndrome (CFS), a condition in which a severe form of unexplained chronic weariness is associated with body pain and other symptoms. Reported in the August 11, 2003 issue of the *Archives of Internal Medicine*, this study of 297 patients by Alexander C. Chester, MD found that most CFS patients also had sinus symptoms. Sinus symptoms were nine times more common in patients with unexplained CFS than in patients with fatigue explained by a mental or physical illness. Chester suggested that more research was necessary but the study offered hope that sinus treatments could, in the future, help alleviate both fatigue and pain.

Relationship Between Allergic Rhinitis and Chronic Sinusitis

The fact that up to 80 percent of adults with chronic sinusitis also have allergic rhinitis makes it clear that there is a link between the two conditions. However, the nature of this relationship needs to be further studied. It appears that allergic rhinitis may "prime" a patient for the later development of chronic sinusitis, but this hypothesis needs to be further evaluated and tested. The question then remains how the two diseases interrelate and what can be done to stop the development of chronic sinusitis. If rhinitis does "prime" an individual toward chronic sinusitis, we need to evaluate whether allergy management in early younger life changes the likelihood of chronic sinusitis in later life.

Connection Between Asthma and Chronic Sinusitis

Similarly, up to 75 percent of those with asthma also get sinusitis. What the link is between these two diseases remains of great interest to both pulmonologists and otolaryngologists. The current evidence would appear to suggest that they are part of the same disease process, and that chronic rhinitis can really be considered an "asthma of the nose." However, it is clear that when chronic sinusitis flares up, it also aggravates asthma in the bronchial airways.

Summary

In summary, chronic rhinosinusitis it is a very common disorder that affects millions of Americans and can be very debilitating, both in terms of time lost from work and quality of life. There is still a great deal of research to be done to identify more about the inflammatory process involved in chronic rhinosinusitis, and about what can be done to prevent it and optimally treat it. It is clear that it is not just a simple bacterial infection, but involves other aspects of the inflammatory process. It also appears that there are factors that may predispose certain people toward sinusitis in the environment, such as smoking and pollution. Allergies and genetic predispositions present in an individual may also make them more susceptible to chronic rhinosinusitis, and local nasal problems, such as a deviated nasal septum, may make symptoms worse, too.

We hope that the information provided in this book will help people avoid the problems caused by this disease, and help those that do have chronic rhinosinusitis manage it, thus ameliorating the impact it has on their lives. We also hope that this book will provide impetus for those who read it to advocate for more research into this common and debilitating disorder, and to do what they can to support research into both its underlying causes and its optimal treatment, so that our children and grandchildren will be free of this chronic problem.

GLOSSARY

ACUTE SINUSITIS Short-lived, episode sinusitis with sudden onset

ADENOIDS Structures made of lymph tissue that lie within the nasopharynx

ALLERGY Hypersensitivity or reaction of the immune system to allergens

ALTERNATIVE MEDICINE Remedies such as herbs and food supplements that are used to treat the symptoms of diseases

ANALGESIC Medication used to treat pain (and sometimes fever)

ANTIBIOTIC Medication used to treat diseases caused by bacteria

ANTIHISTAMINE Medication used to treat allergies which blocks the action of histamine

ASTHMA Disorder characterized by intermittent airway constriction

BACTERIA Single-celled organisms that can cause infections

CHRONIC SINUSITIS Sinusitis that lasts for at least 12 weeks

CILIA Microscopic hairs on the surface of the sinus membranes that provide a sweeping action to move mucus out of the sinuses

COMMON COLD Viral infection of the upper respiratory tract

CONCHA   (See *turbinate*)

CONCHA BULLOSA   A deformity characterized by air-filled middle turbinates

CORTICOSTEROID   Anti-inflammatory medications that are synthetic versions of hormones produced in the body

CYSTIC FIBROSIS   Congenital disorder that results in production of large amounts of thickened mucus

DECONGESTANT   Medications that clear nasal passages of congestion

ETHMOID SINUSES   Sinuses located behind the bridge of the nose between the eyes

FUNCTIONAL ENDOSCOPIC SINUS SURGERY (FESS)   Surgery that uses an endoscope to remove blockages in the ostiomeatal complex and preserves the mucosal lining

FUNGI   Plantlike organisms including mushrooms and molds

FRONTAL SINUSES   Sinuses located over the eyes

IMAGE-GUIDED SURGERY   Surgical technique that uses interactive three-dimensional computer mapping

INFLUENZA   Viral infection of the respiratory tract

INVASIVE SURGERY   Surgery that requires an incision through the skin

LARYNX   Voice box

MAXILLARY SINUSES   Sinuses located inside the cheekbones

MIDDLE MEATUS   Drainage pathway for the ostiomeatal complex

MUCUS   Substance composed of mucins and inorganic salts suspended in water. Mucus is also a component of saliva, and coats the respiratory, gastrointestinal, and genital tracts

MUCOUS MEMBRANE   The delicate lining of the nose and sinuses which secretes mucus

MUCOCILIARY BLANKET   Continuous layer of mucus that coats the cells that line the nose and sinuses

OSTIOMEATAL COMPLEX   The drainage area for the maxillary sinus, frontal sinus, and the anterior ethmoid sinus, on each side

OSTIUM   Opening point at which each sinus empties into the nasal cavity

OTITIS MEDIA   Infection in the inner ear

OTOLARYNGOLOGIST   Specialist in diseases of the ears, nose, and throat

PHARYNX   Part of the throat between the tonsils and the larynx

RECURRENT SINUSITIS   Repeated incidences of sinusitis

RHINITIS   Inflammation of the nose

RHINOSCOPY   An examination of the nose and sinuses using a flexible or rigid endoscope; also known as sinus endoscopy

RHINOSINUSITIS   A more recent term used to recognize that inflammation of the nose and sinuses almost always occur together

SEPTUM   Vertical bone that separates the right and left sides of the nose

SEPTOPLASTY   Surgical procedure to straighten the nasal septum

SPHENOID SINUSES   Sinuses located behind the ethmoid sinuses in the upper nose area behind the eyes

SINUSITIS   Inflammation of the sinuses passages

TONSILS   Clumps of lymph tissue located on both sides of the throat

TURBINATE   Normal structure within the nasal cavity that helps humidify and filter air as it passes through the nose; also known as a concha

VIRUSES   Microscopic organisms that cause diseases such as colds and influenza

SELECTED
BIBLIOGRAPHY

CHAPTER ONE:

American Academy of Otolaryngology, Fact Sheet, *20 Questions about Your Sinuses*, www.entnet.org/healthinfo/sinus/sinus_questions.cfm, March 17, 2003.

National Center for Health Statistics, Centers for Disease Control, *Chronic Sinusitis*, www.cdc.gov/hchs/fastats/sinuses.htm.

Healthy Sinus Anatomy, www.sinusinfocenter.com/images/NormalSinusFrotalView.jpg, March 20, 2003.

Hwang, Peter, M.D., *What are the Common Causes of Sinusitis?*, www.sinusinfocenter.com/stripcontent.php?parent_file=/sinus_faq-02.html, March 20, 2003.

Kennedy, Elicia, M.D., *Sinusitis*, eMedicine, www.emedicine.com/EMERG/topic536.htm.

Mucus and Mucins, arbl.cvmbs.colostate.edu/hbooks/molecules/mucins.html, March 17, 2003.

National Institute of Allergy and Infectious Diseases, *Sinusitis*, www.niaid.hih.gov/factsheets/sinusitis.htm.

Osguthrope, J. David, M.D., *Adult Rhinosinusitis: Diagnosis and Management*, American Family Physician, www.aafp.org/afp/2010101/69.html, March 20, 2003.

Porter, Glen, M.D., *Paranasal Sinus Anatomy and Function*, www.utmb.edu.otoref/Grnds/Paranasal-Sinus-2002-01/Paranasal-sinus-2002-01.htm, March 20, 2003.

Reckert-Reusing, Sandy, *Sinusitis, Nothing to Sneeze At*, Johns Hopkins Bayview Medical Center, www.jhbmc.jhu.edu/OPA/baynews/sp1997/sinus.thml, March 17, 2003.

Sinusitis, www.mamashealth.com/allergies/sinusitis.asp, March 17, 2003.

Sinus Anatomy, www.sinusinfocenter.com/sinus_anatomy.html, March 19, 2003.

Sinusitis Defined, www.sinusinfectioncenter.com, March 20, 2003.

CHAPTER TWO

About the Sinuses, Your Medical Source, www.your medicalsource.com/library/endosinus/ESS_sinuses.html, March 25, 2003.

Adenoids and Adenoidectomy, Texas Pediatric Surgical Associates, www.pedisurg.com/pPtEducENT/adenoids.htm, March 26, 2003

Anatomy and Function of the Nose, www.entlink.net.education/curriculum/nose_anat_func.cfm, March 23, 2003

Anatomy and Physiology of the Paranasal Sinuses, www.entlink.net/education/curricullum/sinusanat.cfm, March 20, 2003.

Anatomy of the Paranasal Sinuses, Rad Sci Online, www.radscice.com/5611b.html, Citardi, Martin J., M.D., *Brief Overview of Sinus and Nasal Anatomy*, American Rhinologic Society, american-rhinologic.org, March 17, 2003.

Diagram of the Eye, National Eye Institute, www.nei.hih.gov/health/ eyediagram/index.thm, March 26, 2003.

Diseases of the Ear, Nose and Throat, The Nose and the Paranasal Sinuses, Columbia University College of P&S Complete Home Medical Guide, www.cpmcnet.columbia.edu/texts/guide/ hmg31_0009.thml, March 26, 2003.

Ear Anatomy, www.enchantedlearning.com/subjects/anatomy/ ear/, March 26, 2003.

Everything You Always Wanted to Know about Noses, www. wcsscience.com/nose/page.html, March 26, 2003.

Eye Anatomy, St. Luke's Cataract & Laser Institute, www. stlukeseye.com/Anatomy.asp, March 26, 2003

Human Respiratory System, American Lung Association, www.lungusa.org/learn/resp_sys.html, March 20, 2003.

Organ Delivery System, www.sln.fi.edu/biosci/systems/ respiration.html, March 20, 2003.

Porter, Glen, M.D., Paranasal *Sinus Anatomy and Function*, www.utmb.edu.otoref/Grnds/Paranasal-Sinus-2002-01/ Paranasal-sinus-2002-01.htm, March 20, 2003.

The Parts of the Eye, www.cis.rit.edu/people/faculty/montag/ vandplite/pages/chap_9/ch9p3.thml, March 26, 2003.

Respiratory System: Structure Detail, American Medical Association, www.ama-assn.org/ama/pub/category/7166.html, March 20, 2003.

Respiratory System, www.biology.clc.uc.edu/courses/bio105/ respirat.htm, March 20, 2003.

Review of Anatomy: Nose and Paranasal Sinuses, The Bobby R. Alford
   Department of Otorhinolaryngology and Communicative
   Sciences, Baylor College of Medicine, www.bcm.tmc.edu/oto/
   studs/anat/nose.html, March 23, 2003.

Rosin, Deborah, M.D., *The Sinuses—What They Are and What
   They Do*, WebMD, www.webmd.lycos.com/content/article/7/
   1680_51928?UID=%7B308A5FA9-C77F-44B)-B, March 25,
   2003.

Salivary Glands and Saliva, www.arbl.cvmbs.colostate.edu/hbooks/
   pathphys/digestion/pregastric/salivary.html, March 26, 2003.

Sinus Anatomy, Sinus InfoCenter.Com, www.sinusinfocenter.
   com/sinus_anatomy.html, March 19, 2003.

Sinus and Nasal Problems, Florida Ear and Sinus Center, www.earsi-
   nus.com/Brochures/Sinus%20&%20Nasal%20Problems.htm,

CHAPTER THREE

The Body's First Line of Defense, National Institute of Allergy
   and Infectious Diseases, www.niaid.nih.gov/final/immun/
   immun/htm.

Earache, www.warrenclinic.com/housecalls/adult/EarSymptoms/
   Earache.asp, March 13, 2003.

Earache in Children, www.healthsquare.com/mc/fgmc0307.htm,
   March 13, 2003.

Greenberg, Jayson, M.D., *Current Management of Nasal Polyposis*,
   The Bobby R. Alford Department of Otorhinolaryngology
   and Communicative Sciences, www.bcm.tmc.edu/oto/grand/
   090398.html, April 19, 2003.

Sinusitis, National Institute of Allergy and Infectious Diseases, National Institutes of Health, www.niaid.nih.gov/factsheets/ sinusitis.htm, April 19, 2003.

CHAPTER FOUR

What is an Otolaryngologist, American Academy of Otolaryngology— Head and Neck Surgery, www.entnet.org/healthinfo/about/ otolaryngologist.cfm.

CHAPTER FIVE

Adult Rhinosinusitis: Diagnosis and Management, American Family Physician, www.aafp.org/afp/20010101/69.html, March 20, 2003.

Anand, Vijay K., M.D., *Radiologic Imaging Studies,* www.sinusitis-solutions.com/radiologic.html.

Citardi, Martin J., M.D., *An Introduction to Nasal Endoscopy,* American Rhinologic Society, www.american-rhinologic.org/ cgi-bin/menu.cgi?m=main.menu&state=10011255551000000, March 17, 2003.

The Common Cold, National Institute of Allergy and Infectious Diseases, National Institutes of Health, www.niaid.hih.gov/ factsheets/cold.htm, May 22, 2003.

CT scan, Netdoctor.co.uk, www.netdoctor.co.ukhealth_advice/ examinations/ctgenreal.htm, March 14, 2003.

CT (Cat) Scan: Brief History of CT, St. Michael's Hospital, www.stmichaelshospital.com/content/programs/medical_ imaging/ct_scan/ct_history.asp, May 15, 2003.

Gum Diseases, www.dentalpath.com/dp/dp_dg.htm, May 22, 2003.

The History of MRI, Ensil International Corp, www.ensil.com/
    Database/DB-Medical/Dmed-History%20of%20MRI.html,
    May 15, 2003.

How MRI Works, www.howstuffworks.com/mri/htm, May 15, 2003.

How is Sinusitis Diagnosed?, Michigan Sinus Center,
    www.med.umich.edu/oto/misinus/faqs/pgthree.htm,
    May 14, 2003.

Influenza: The Disease, National Center for Infectious Diseases,
    www.cdc.gov/ncidod/diseases/flu/fluinfo.htm, May 22, 2003.

The Migraine Relief Center, www.migrainehelp.com/understand/
    causes.html, May 22, 2003.

A Short History of Magnetic Resonance from a European Point of View,
    www.emrf.org/FAQs%20MRI%20History.html, May 15, 2003.

Sinus X-ray for Sinusitis, www.informationtherapy.org/kbase/topic/
    detail/test/hw60323/detail.htm, May 14, 2003.

Sinusitis, www.healthandage.com/Home/gm=6!gid6=6206,
    May 15, 2003.

Sinusitis, National Institute of Allergy and Infectious Diseases,
    www.niaid, hih.gov/factsheets/sinusitis.htm, March 17, 2003.

Temporomandibular Disorder (TMD), University of Maryland
    Medicine, www.umm.edu/oralhealth/tmd.htm, May 27, 2003.

What is Trigeminal Neuralgia?, Trigeminal Neuralgia Association,
    www.tna_support.org/Definition.htm, May 22, 2003.

CHAPTER SIX

Acute Sinusitis, MayoClinic.com, www.mayoclinic.com/invoke.
dfm?id=DS00170, March 27, 2003.

Acute sinusitis, www.acutesinusitis.com/sinusfacts.html, March 27,
2003.

Anand, Vijay K., M.D., *What is Recurrent Sinusitis?*,
www.sinusitis-solutions.com/revision.html, March 27, 2003.

Meningitis, MayoClinic.com, www.mayoclinic.com/invoke/
cfm?id=DS00118, March 27, 2003.

Sinusitis Overview, Sinus Pharmacy, www.sinuspharmacy.com/
sinusitis.html, August 11, 2003.

CHAPTER SEVEN

About the Sinuses, Your Medical Source, www.yourmedical
source.com/library/endosinus/ESS_sinuses.html, March 25,
2003.

Arkangel, Carmelito, Jr., M.D., *Cocaine Abuse*,
www.emedicine.com/aaem/topic112.htm, March 28, 2003.

Bacteria, www.microbe.org/microbes/bacterium1.asp, March 28,
2003.

Causes, Health Care Information for Sinus Sufferers, Sinus
InfoCenter.com, www.sinusinfocenter.com, March 17, 2003.

Chronic Nasal Obstruction/Your Stuffy Nose, Department of
Otolaryngology/Head and Neck Surgery, Columbia University,
www.entcolumbia.org/nasobst.htm, March 28, 2003.

Cystic Fibrosis, National Center for Biotechnology Information, www.ncbi.nlm.hih.gov/books/bv.fcgi?call=bv.View, March 28, 2003.

Definition of Infection, www.gruenthal.com/wwwgrt/template/all/service/knowledgebase/antibiotica/content_, March 28, 2003.

Fungal Sinusitis, American Academy of Otolaryngology Head and Neck Surgery, www.entnet.org/healthinfo/sinus/fungal_sinusitis.cfm, March 17, 2003.

Gene Alterations for Cystic Fibrosis May Also Account for Chronic Sinus Problems in Some, National Institute of Allergy and Infectious Diseases, www.sciencedaily.com/releases/2000/10/001011071550.htm, March 28, 2003.

Greenberg, Jayson, M.D., *Current Management of Nasal Polyposis*, Bobby R. Alford Department of Otolaryngology and Communicative Sciences, www.bcm.tmc.edu/oto/grand/090398.html, March 23, 2003.

Hwang, M.D., *What is a Concha Bullosa?*, SinusInfoCenter.com, www.sinusinfocenter.com/stripcontent.pho?parent_file+/sinus_faq_08.html, March 28, 2003.

Immotile Cilia Syndrome, www.asthma.about.com/library/weekly/aa090400a.htm, March 28, 2003.

McKean, Laury, R.N., *Sinusitis & HIV*, Seattle Treatment Education Project, www.aegis.com/pubs/step/1993/STEP5120.html,

Nasal Polyps, New York Allergy and Sinus Centers, www.nyallergy.com/Conditions/nasal_polyps.htm, March 28, 2003.

Reflux Disease May Cause Sinusitis and Damage Teeth, HealthLink, Medical College of Wisconsin, www.healthlink.mcw.edu/article/968784529.html, March 28, 2003.

Sinusitis, Health.com, www.health.com/health/wynks/
   SinusisitWYNK2000-MAL/causes.html, March 28, 2003.

Sinusitis, www.mothernature.com/Library/bookshelf/Books/62/
   84.cfm, March 28, 2003.

Viral Infections, The Merck Manual, www.merck.com/
   mrkshared/mmanual_home/sce17/186.jsp, March 28, 2003.

What Causes a Bacterial Infection? Health A to Z, www.
   healthatoz.com/healthatoz/Atoz/dc/caz/infc/bact/baccause.htm
   l, March 28, 2003.

CHAPTER EIGHT

Acari, www.sel.barc.usda.gov/acari/content/watermite/
   rotate.html, March 26, 2003.

Allergy, Allergic Disease, Allergic Disorders, Allergic Illness, Health on the
   Net Foundation, www.hon.ch/Library/Theme/Allergy/
   Glossary/allergy.html, March 26, 2003.

Allergies and Hay Fever, American Academy of Otolaryngology Head
   and Neck Surgery, www.entnet.org.healthinfo/allergies/
   allergies_hayfever.cfm, March 27, 2003.

Asthma, Health on the Net Foundation, www.hon.ch/Library/
   Theme/Allergy/Glossary/asthma.html, March 26, 2003.

Asthma, www.radix.net/~mwg/triggers.html, March 26, 2003.

Colds & Flu, The American Academy of Family Physicians,
   www.quickcare.org/resp/colds/html, March 26, 2003.

Deviated Septum, Otolaryngology Head and Neck Surgery,
   Johns Hopkins Otolaryngology, www.hopkinsmedicine.org/
   otolaryngology/disorders/other/deviated.html, March 27, 2003.

Drug Allergies, Medline Health Information, www.nlm.hih.gov/medlineplus/ency/article/00919.htm, March 26, 2003.

Exercise-Induced Asthma, www.emedicine.com/sports/byname/ exercise-induced-asthma.htm, August 15, 2003.

Fact Sheet: Allergic Rhinitis, Sinusitis and Rhionsinusitis, American Academy of Otolaryngology Head and Neck Surgery, www. entnet.org/healthinfo/sinus/allergic_rhinitis.cfm, March 17, 2003.

Facts About Asthma, American Lung Association, www.lungusa.org/asthma/astasthma/html, March 26, 2003.

Influenza: The Disease, National Center for Infectious Disease, Centers for Disease Control, www.dcd.gov/ncidod/diseases/ flu/fluinfo.htm, March 27, 2003.

1918 Influenza Pandemic, www.stanford.edu/group/virus/uda, March 27, 2003.

Pirquet, Clemens, Baron von, www.cartage.org.lb/en/themes/ Biographies/MainBiographies/P/Pirquet/1.html, April 9, 2003.

Q&A: Severe Acute Respiratory Syndrome (SARS), www.cnn.com/ 2003/HEALTH/03/27/illness.qa, April 9, 2003.

Severe Acute Respiratory Syndrome (SARS)—multi-country outbreak—Update 24, World Health Organization, www.who.int/csr/don/2003_04_08/en/, April 9, 2003.

Sinus Facts: An Overview, Sinus News, www.sinusnews.com/ Articles/sinus-facts-overview.html, August 15, 2003.

Vasomotor Rhinitis, Healthlink, Medical College of Wisconsin, www.healthlink.mcw.edu/article/899250622.html, March 27, 2003.

Vasomotor Rhinitis, National Headache Foundation, www.headaches. org/consumer/topicsheets/Vasomotorrhinitis.html, March 27, 2003.

What are NSAIDs?, Your Orthopaedic Connection, American Academy of Orthopaedic Surgeons, www.orthoinfo.aaos.com, August 15, 2003.

CHAPTER NINE

Acute sinusitis, www.MayoClinic.com/invoke/crm?id=DS00170, May 28, 2003.

Cancers of the Nose and the Paranasal Sinuses, www.indaicancer. org/coca/n/nasal/html, March 25, 2003.

Intracranial Complications of Sinusitis, Sinus News, www.sinusnews. comArticles2/intracranialsinusitis.html, May 28, 2003.

Inverting Papilloma, Paranasal Sinus, www.eu.amershamhealth.com/ medcyclopaedia/Volume%20VII/INVERTING%20PAPILLO, May 28, 2003.

Lethal Midline Granuloma, www.amershamhealth.com/ medcyclopaedia/Volume%20VI202/lethal%20midline%2, May 28, 2003.

Meningitis, www.MayoClinic.com/invoke.cfm?id=DS00118, May 28, 2003.

Periostitis, www.amershamhealth.com/medcyclopaedia/Volume% 20III%201/Periostititis.asp, March 17, 2003.

Septicemia, Medline Health Information, www.nlm.nih.gov/ medlineplus/ency/article/001355.htm, March 17, 2003.

Shah, Nishit J., *Complications of Sinusitis*, Bombay Hospital Journal, Bombay Hospital and Medical Research Centre, www.bhy.org/journal/1999_4104_oct99/sp_642.htm, March 17, 2003.

Sinus Mucoceles Defined, Sinus News, January 1, 2002, www.sinusnews.com/Articles/sinus-mucoceles-defined.html, March 29, 2003.

The Nose and the Paranasal Sinuses, www.cpmcnet.columbia.edu/ texts/guide/hmg31_009l.html, March 26, 2003.

What Is Melanoma?, www.melanoma.com/melanoma, May 28, 2003.

What Is Sarcoma?, www.sarcoma.net/facts.htm, May 28, 2003.

CHAPTER TEN

Nasal Sprays: How to Use them Correctly, www.familydoctor.org/ handouts/104.html, March 17, 2003.

How to Use a Steroid Nasal Spray, St. John's Mercy Hospital, www.stjohnsmercy.org/mmg/mmghealthinfo/adults/allergiesast hma/howtousespray.asp, March 17, 2003.

CHAPTER ELEVEN

Antihistamines, Decongestants and Cold Remedies, American Academy of Otolaryngology—Head and Neck Surgery, www.entnet.org/ healthinfo/allergies/antihistamines.cfm, March 17, 2003.

Casano, Peter J., M.D., *Sinusitis and Over-the-Counter Meds*, www.sinuscarecenter.com/otc_aao.html, September 19, 2003.

Fact Sheet: Antibiotics and Sinusitis, American Academy of Otolaryngology—Head and Neck Surgery, www.entnet.org/ healthinfo/sinus/antibiotics_sinusitis.cfm, March 17, 2003.

Fact Sheet: Sinus Pain—Can Over-the-Counter Medications Help?, American Academy of Otolaryngology—Head and Neck Surgery, www.entnet.org/heatlhinfo/sinus/sinus_pain.cfm, March 17, 2003.

History of Antibiotics, www.molbio.princeton.edu/courses/
    mb427/2001/projects/02/antibiotics.htm, May 15, 2003.

Holten, Keith B., M.D. and Edward M. Onusko, M.D., *Appropriate
    Prescribing of Oral Beta-Lactam Antibiotics,* American Family
    Physician, August 1, 2000, www.aafp.org.afp/20000801/
    611.html, November 19, 2003.

McKean, Laury, RN, *Sinusitis & HIV*, www.aegis.com/pubs/
    step/1993/STEPS5120.thml, March 28, 2003.

Microbes: What Doesn't Kill Them Makes Them Stronger, www.
    whyfiles.org/038badbugs/scope.html, September 29, 2003.

Steroid Nasal Sprays Seem to Speed Sinusitis Recovery, Duke
    University Medical Center, www.sciencedaily.com/releases/
    2001/12/011227074737.htm, March 19, 2003.

Sinusitis, www.healthandage.com/Home/gm=6!gid6=6209,
    May 15, 2003.

What Causes a Bacterial Infection?, Health AtoZ, www.healthatoz.
    com/healthatoz/Atoz/dc/caz/infc/bact/baccause.html.

CHAPTER TWELVE

Martin, Lawrence, M.D., FACP, FCCP, *Cough, Chronic Cough, Rhini-
    tis and Sinusitis— a Table of Drugs*, www.mtsinai.org/
    pulmonary/Cough/drugs.htm, September 19, 2003.

What Are the Medications for Chronic or Recurrent Sinusitis?,
    University of Maryland Medicine, www.umn.edu/patiented/
    articles/what_medications_chronic_or_recurrentsinusitis_00,
    September 18, 2003.

CHAPTER THIRTEEN

Endoscopic Sinus Surgery, Your Medical Source, www.your
   medicalsource.com/library/endosinus.html, March 25, 2003.

Kennedy, D. W., M.D., *Sinus Surgery: A Century of Controversy*, Laryngoscope, 105:1, pp. 1-5, January 1997.

Kennedy, D. W., M.D., S. J. Zinreich, A. E. Rosenbaum, M. Johns.
   *Functional Endoscopic Sinus Surgery: Theory and Diagnostic Evalua-
   tion*, Arch Oto 111: , pp. 576-582, September 1985.

Kennedy, D. W., M.D., S. J. *The Functional Endoscopic Approach to
   Inflammatory Sinus Disease: Current Perspectives and Technique
   Modifications*, Am. J. Rhinol. 2:3, pp. 89-96, Summer 1988.

Zinreich, S. J., S. A. Tebo, D. M. Long, H. Brem, D. E. Mattox,
   M. E. Loury, C. A. Vander Colk, W. M. Koch, D. W. Kennedy, R.
   N. Bryan. *Frameless Stereotaxic Integration of CT Imaging Data:
   Accuracy and Initial Applications.* Radiology, 188:3, pp. 735-742,
   September 1993.

Kennedy, D. W., W. Boger, S. J. Zinreich. *Diseases of the Sinuses, Diagnosis and Management*, BC Decker, Hamilton, 2001.

Lanza, D. C., D. A. O'Brien, D. W. Kennedy. *Endoscopic Repair of Cerebrospinal Fluid Fistulae in Encephaloceles*, Laryngoscope, 106:9,
   pp 1119-1125, September 1996.

CHAPTER FOURTEEN

Adenoid Removal, Medline Health Information, www.nlm.nih.
   gov/medlineplus/ency/article/003011.htm, March 17, 2003.

Fact Sheet: Deviated Septum, American Academy of Otolaryngology—Head and Neck Surgery, www.entnet.org/healthinfo/
sinus/deviated-septem.cfm, March 27, 2003.

Fact Sheet: Sinus Surgery, American Academy of Otolaryngology—
Head and Neck Surgery, www.entnet.org/healthinfo/sinus/
sinus_surgery.cfm, March 17, 2003.

Whitaker, Elizabeth, M.D., *Rhinoplasty, Turbinate Reduction*,
eMedicine, www.emedicine.com/;lastic/topic101.htm,
March 20, 2003.

CHAPTER FIFTEEN

Center for Drug Evaluation and Research, www.fda.gov.cder/
warn/cyber/2002/DRSANallnatherb.htm, September 18, 2002.

Dragon, Victoria, *Acupressure for Sinusitis*, www/acupuncture.
com/TuiNa/sinus.htm, March 17, 2003.

Evans, Mark, *Natural Healing: Remedies & Therapies*, Hermes House,
London, 2001.

Hoffman, David L., B.Sc. (Hons), MNIMH, *Sinusitis*, www.healthy.
net.asp/templates/article.asp?PageType=article&ID=1610,
March 17, 2003.

Kapadia, Manish, *Homeopathy for Sinusitis*, www.healthlibrary.
com/reading/yod/dec/chapt4.htm, March 19, 2003.

Natural Medicines & Homeopathy, Arnica.com, www.arnica.com/
tips/tip5/html, November 16, 2001.

Medical Advisor, The, *The Complete Guide to Alternative &
Conventional Treatments*, Time Life Books, New York, 1996.

Natural Therapeutics, Health World Online, www.healthy.net/asp/
templates/article.asp?PageTy;e=Article&ID=7, February 6, 2002.

Rosenfeld, Idadore, M.D., *Dr. Rosenfeld's Guide to Alternative Medicine*, Random House, New York, 1996.

Sinusitis, AltHealth.co.uk, www.althealth.co.uk/services/info/ ailments/sinusitis1.pho, September 18, 2003.

Sinusitis, Nature Cure, www.healthlibrary.com/reading/ncure/ chapt76.htm, March 17, 2003.

Spices, Spice Seeds and Herbs, U.S. Food and Drug Administration, www.fda.gov/opacom/morechoices/smallbusiness/blubook/spic es.htm, September 18, 2002.

Supplements, Wholehealthmd.com, www.wholehealthmd.com/ref-shelf/subs...?0,1525,10040,00.thm, November 6, 2002.

Walkinshaw, Catharine, *What is Reiki?* www.eatonville.com/ walkinshaw/health5.thml, February 6, 2002.

Williams, Thom, Ph.D., *The Complete Illustrated Guide to Chinese Medicine*, Element, Rockport, MA, 1996.

CHAPTER SIXTEEN

Allergies and Hay Fever: Insight into Causes, Treatment and Prevention, American Academy of Otolaryngology—Head and Neck Surgery, www.entnet.org/healthinfo/allergies/allergies_ hayfever.cfm, March 17, 2003.

Preventing Future Sinus Problems, Your Medical Source, www.yourmedicalsource.com/library/endosinus/ESS_prevent.ht ml, March 25, 2003.

Sinusitis Prevention, Personal Health Zone, www.personalhealth zone.com/sinusitis_prevention.html, March 17, 2003.

Therapeutics: Environmental Controls, Johns Hopkins Asthma & Allergy, www.hopkins-allergy.org/sinusitis/therapeutics-house.html, March 17, 2003.

CHAPTER EIGHTEEN

Fact Sheet: Sinusitis: Special Considerations for Aging Patients, American Academy of Otolaryngology—Head and Neck Surgery, www.entnet.org/healthinfo/sinus/aging_patients.cfm, October 16, 2003.

Henig, Noreen, M.D.*, Sinusitis and Cystic Fibrosis,* www.cfcenter. stanford.edu/CFNews-Sinusitis.htm, October 16, 2003.

Pregnancy and Sinusitis, www.sinusinfocenter.com/sinus_causes_lifestyle.html, October 16, 2003.

Sinusitis in Children, Department of Otolaryngology/Head and Neck Surgery, Columbia University, www.entcolumbia.org/sininf.htm, October 16, 2003.

Who Gets Sinusitis?, University of Maryland Medicine, www.umm. edu/patiented/articles/who_gets_sinusitis_000062_3.htm, October 16, 2003.

Wilson, William R., *Nose and Throat Disorders,* The Merck Manual of Geriatrics, www.merck.com/pubs/mm_geriatrics/sec15/ch130.htm, October 16, 2003.

CHAPTER NINETEEN

Aerosolized Antibiotics Prove to Be Safe and Effective Treatment for Sinusitis, www.sinusitiscenter.com/Studies/aerosolized_antibiotics. html, October 16, 2003.

Diagnosing Chronic Fatigue? Check for Sinusitis, ScienceDaily News Release, www.sciencedaily.com/releases/2003/08/030814072847.htm, October 16, 2003.

Efficacy and Tolerability of Cefprozil versus Amoxicillin/clavulanate for the Treatment of Adults with Severe Sinusitis, Clinical Therapies, November–December 1998, 20:6, pp. 1115-1129.

Enzyme May Play Unexpected Role in Asthma, www.sinusitis center.com?News/enzyme_asthma.html, October 16, 2003.

Gene Alterations for Cystic Fibrosis May Also Account for Chronic Sinus Problems in Some, National Institute of Alllergy and Infectious Diseases, www.sciencedaily.com/releases/2000/10/0010110 71550.htm,

Hopkins Researchers Uncover Sinus Infection-CF Gene Link, www.sci-encedaily.com/releases/2000/10/001009104808.htm, October 16, 2003.

Mayo Clinic Study Implicates Fungus as Cause of Chronic Sinusitis, www.sciencedaily.com/releases/1999/09/990910080344.htm, October 16, 2003.

Nebulized Antibiotics, www.sinusitiscentral.com/nebulized_antibiotics.html, October 16, 2003.

New Therapy May Ease Stubborn Sinusitis, wwwl.excite.com/home/health/health_article/0,11720,511547,00.html, March 17, 2003.

Sinusitis Linked to Chronic Fatigue, www.Sinuscenter.com/News/chronic_fatigue.html, October 16, 2003.

Study Provides Research Essential to Development of Medication for Loss of Smell, www.sinusitiscenter.com/Studies/loss_of_smell.html, October 16, 2003.

What Research Is Going On? National Institutes of Health, www.niaid.hih.gov/factsheets/sinusitis.htm, October 16, 2003.

RESOURCES

Organizations

AMERICAN ACADEMY OF OTOLARYNGOLOGY—HEAD AND NECK
SURGERY, INC.
One Prince Street
Alexandria, VA 22314
(703) 836-4444
www.entnet.org

AMERICAN RHINOLOGIC SOCIETY
Montefieore Medical Center
Department of Otolaryngology
3400 Bainbridge Avenue
MAP 3rd Floor
Bronx, NY 10467
www.american-rhinologic.org

AMERICAN ACADEMY OF ALLERGY, ASTHMA AND IMMUNOLOGY
611 E. Wells Street
Milwaukee, WI 53202
(800) 822-ASMA (2762)
www.aaaai.org

ASTHMA AND ALLERGY FOUNDATION OF AMERICA (AAFA)
  1233 20th Street, Suite 402
  Washington, DC 20036
  (202) 466-7643
  (800) 7-Asthma
  www.aafa.org

CENTER FOR CURRENT RESEARCH, INC.
  706 Aubrey Avenue
  Ardmore, PA 19003
  (610) 649-3166
  www.lifestages.com

CYSTIC FIBROSIS FOUNDATION
  6931 Arlington Road
  Bethesda, MD 20814
  (301) 951-6378
  www.cff.org

JOINT COUNCIL OF ALLERGY, ASTHMA AND IMMUNOLOGY
  50 N. Brockway, Suite 3.3
  Palatine, IL 60067
  (847) 934-1918
  www.jcaai.org

NATIONAL INSTITUTE OF ALLERGY AND INFECTIOUS DISEASES
  Building 31, Room 7A-50
  31 Center Drive MSC 2520
  Bethesda, MD 20892
  www.hiaid.hih.gov.

Other Books About Sinusitis

Bruce, Debra Fulghum, Murray Grossan, MD, *The Sinus Cure: 7 Simple Steps to Relieve Sinusitis and Other Ear, Nose and Throat Conditions*, Ballantine Books, New York, 2001.

Plasse, Harvey, MD, Shelagh Ryan Masline, *Sinusitis Relief*, Henry Holt and Company, LLC, New York, 2002.

Rosin, Deborah F., MD, *The Sinus Sourcebook*, Lowell House, Los Angeles, 1998.

Williams, M. Lee, MD, *The Sinusitis Help Book*, John Wiley and Sons, New York, 1998.

INDEX

A

Absent cilia, 77
Accolate®, 149
Accupressure, 188
Acetaminophen, 110, 136, 148
Actifed®, 148
Acupuncture, 187–188
Acute bacterial rhinosinusitis, 70
Acute rhinosinusitis, 63, 120
Acute sinusitis, 240
Adenocarcinoma, 106
Adenoidectomy, 177–178
Adenoids, 23, 53, 83–84, 240
Adenoviruses, 46
Advil®, 110, 135
Aesthetic nasal surgery, 176
Afrin®, 104, 146, 224
Air conditioners, 203
Air pollution, effects of, 73–74
Air travel, 211–212
Airplane flights, 84–85
Aleve®, 135, 224
Allegra®, 147, 148
Allergic fungal rhinosinusitis, 71–72
Allergic rhinitis and chronic sinusitis, relationship between, 238
Allergic rhinosinusitis, 3
Allergic shiners, 31
Allergies, 48–49, 74, 87–88, 89, 109, 205–207, 240
Allergies, treating patients with rhinosinusitis and, 121–122
Allergy desensitization, 109, 122, 208–209

Allergy testing, 208–209
Altenaria, 202
Alternative medicine
    accupressure, 188
    acupuncture, 187–188
    applications of, 184–186
    aromatherapy, 193
    availability of, 191
    Chinese medicine, 186–187
    consulting your doctor, 197
    dietary remedies, 194–195
    direct action of, 191
    dosage, 191
    food supplements, 193–194, 195–196
    herbal medicines, 193–194
    herbal remedies, 194
    homeopathy, 188–189
    Internet, obtaining drugs from the, 196
    naturopathy, 189–190
    origin of mainstream medicine, 182–183
    precautions for, 213–214
    prescientific medicinal theories, 181–182
    purity, issues of, 190–191
    regulation of, 192
    renewed interest in, 183–184
    side effects, 191–192
Amoxicillin-clavulanate, 137
Amoxil®, 137, 225
Ampicillin sodium, 137
Analgesics, 135–136, 240
Analysis of your symptoms, completing an, 44–45

T

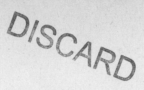

HEALTHY LIVING BOOKS

Healthy Living Books brings together recognized experts from the fields of health, medicine, fitness, and nutrition to provide millions of men and women with the reliable information they need to lead longer, healthier lives.

Our editors recognize that good health comes from healthy lifestyle choices: eating well, exercising regularly, and preventing illness through sound knowledge and intelligent action.

In this day and age, when fewer people are covered by health insurance and more face increased health risks due to sedentary lifestyles, improper nutrition, and the challenges of aging, there is a profound need for solid, tested guidance. That's where we fit in.

Our medical team consists of physicians and specialists from the country's leading medical centers and institutions. Our recipes are kitchen-tested for reliability and include nutritional analysis so that home cooks will find it easy to put delicious, healthful meals on the table. Our exercise programs are prepared by nationally certified personal trainers and rehabilitation experts. All titles are presented in clear, concise language that makes reading fun and useful.

Visit our Web site at
www.healthylivingbooks.com

Healthy Living Books has something for everyone.